Eat Like a Champion

Performance Nutrition for Your Young Athlete

D0047486

Jill Castle, MS, RDN, CDN

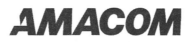

American Management Association
New York • Atlanta • Brussels • Chicago • Mexico City • San Francisco
Shanghai • Tokyo • Toronto • Washington, D. C.

Bulk discounts available. For details visit:
www.amacombooks.org/go/specialsales
Or contact special sales:
Phone: 800-250-5308
Email: specialsls@amanet.org
View all the AMACOM titles at: www.amacombooks.org
American Management Association: www.amanet.org

This publication is designed to provide accurate and authoritative information in regard to the subject matter covered. It is sold with the understanding that the publisher is not engaged in rendering legal, accounting, or other professional service. If legal advice or other expert assistance is required, the services of a competent professional person should be sought.

Library of Congress Cataloging-in-Publication Data

Castle, Jill, 1966-
   Eat like a champion : performance nutrition for your young athlete / Jill Castle, MS, RDN, CDN.
   pages cm
   Includes bibliographical references and index.
   ISBN 978-0-8144-3622-6 (pbk.) — ISBN 0-8144-3622-6 (pbk.) — ISBN 978-0-8144-3623-3 (ebook) — ISBN 0-8144-3623-4 (ebook) 1. Athletes—Nutrition. 2. Teenage athletes—Health and hygiene. I. Title.
   TX361.A8C38 2015
   613.7'11—dc23   2015002871

About AMA
American Management Association (www.amanet.org) is a world leader in talent development, advancing the skills of individuals to drive business success. Our mission is to support the goals of individuals and organizations through a complete range of products and services, including classroom and virtual seminars, webcasts, webinars, podcasts, conferences, corporate and government solutions, business books, and research. AMA's approach to improving performance combines experiential learning—learning through doing—with opportunities for ongoing professional growth at every step of one's career journey.

Printing number

10 9 8 7 6 5 4 3 2

For Gracie, Madeline, Caroline, and Ben:

May you always stay connected to the young athlete who lives inside you.

CONTENTS

PART II PLAY-BY-PLAY EATING

PART III CLEARING THE HURDLES

ACKNOWLEDGMENTS

A book like this doesn't happen by itself. I'd like to thank the many friends, colleagues, and family members who helped me along the way:

To my husband, Jon, who let me set the alarm for 4:30 a.m. most days of the week, and who was ready to be the primary parent when needed. Your unending support and understanding keeps me going.

To my dad, who sparked my interest in nutrition.

To my outstanding research assistant, Leigh Delavan, RD, for her help with this project.

To my registered dietitian colleagues and my family and friends who kindly read portions of this book during its writing. To the dietitians, research experts, and professional athletes who graciously gave their opinions and expertise, and provided quotations used in this book.

And, last, thanks to my terrific agent, Lauren Galit of LKG Agency, who helped make this book a reality, along with Bob Nirkind and the staff at AMACOM Books, who provided guidance and support along the way.

INTRODUCTION

Young athletes need skills, training, mental preparation, and nutrition.
Success doesn't happen when you leave out any one of these.
—Yan Vengerovskiy, head coach and cofounder,
Maritime Rowing Club/New Canaan High School Crew

Sixteen-year-old Ethan, a rising tennis star, found himself in a progressive performance slump. Losing competitions and struggling to get through his regular training schedule, he mistakenly thought a shoulder injury was dragging him down. After months of physical therapy, he went to his pediatrician, who was alarmed by his lack of growth and sent him to me.

Ethan wasn't any taller than he had been at age 14, and his muscles hadn't filled out as expected. Ethan was putting in time and effort to train, day in and day out, including extra weekend lessons. His tennis plateau wasn't from a lack of effort or an insufficient drive to win. It stemmed from a poor diet. Ethan wasn't eating enough, or nutritiously enough, particularly considering the grueling workout he put in each day.

He was skipping breakfast many mornings, eating a protein bar for lunch, and often turning up late for practice after school, when he would eat another protein bar—or not. Ethan usually felt sick to his stomach and fatigued after practice, so when he got home he didn't want to eat dinner. Instead, he ate late at night, after his homework was done and he had showered and relaxed a bit, while talking with his friends on the phone. Then he ate his favorite foods: a whole pizza or a submarine sandwich and chips.

Ethan was making the mistake many young athletes make. He was missing one of the main ingredients for athletic success: solid nutrition. Unfortunately, Ethan's nutrition had been poor for years, and as a result, he wasn't as tall or as muscular as he wanted to be. Ethan needed a big dose of sports nutrition—not only for his athletic endeavors, but for improved growth and his overall health.

Together, we worked to build a solid nutrition plan, which gave him more calories, nutrients, and fluids, balanced throughout his day. I built more structure and timing into his meals and snacks; asked his mom to have a healthy dinner ready when he returned home from practice; and encouraged Ethan to dump the late-night junk foods. I wanted him to make sure he ate breakfast before he left for school, as this would not only interrupt his overnight fast but set the appetite hormones in motion and nourish his body. Packing healthy snacks in his duffel was critical, as he needed to stay on top of eating all day long, not just as an afterthought or when he felt hungry. I also laid out a hydration plan, gave him tips for boosting calories on tournament weekends, and taught him about the role of food in fueling athletic performance.

Eventually, Ethan overcame his tennis plateau, improved his game, gained muscle weight, and had the resources and knowledge to be motivated to eat for both sport and health.

In this book, I will provide a broad background of knowledge for parents of young athletes like Ethan. I'll share information on how and what to eat for optimal athletic performance, showcase the dangers of nutritional imbalances, poor food choices, and improper timing of meals and snacks, and offer insight on how to manage the athlete nutritionally given the challenges that may arise during the childhood and adolescent years. Along the way, I'll try to correct misunderstandings about the relationship of food and eating to optimal athletic performance.

Nutrition Is the Secret Weapon

When you think about youth sports and what separates the top perform-ers from the pack, what comes to mind? Why does one young athlete run faster than everyone around him? Jump higher? Hit the ball farther? Get there first?

Perhaps you think sports success comes from a natural gift or raw talent. Or that it takes large sums of money for lessons, equipment, and performance gear. If you're a coach, you may think athletic success is a direct result of precise technique or more training hours in the gym. If you're a nutritionist, like me, you proclaim the power of food and proper fueling. The truth is, it's all of the above: training, gear, and fueling with good nutrition.

Unfortunately, athletes, parents, and coaches often overlook the im-portance of nutrition for youth sports or misdirect their efforts. Many young athletes don't eat to compete. They're slowed down by fatty, sugary foods, not enough calories, or the wrong (and even dangerous) foods. These poor eating habits can cause them to actually lose in athletic com-petition, and compromise their lifelong health. And like Ethan, some barely meet average annual growth rates.

Some young athletes munch like mini–adult athletes, downing pro-tein shakes and loading up on protein bars. Others eat like toddlers, stick-ing to kiddie food like chicken nuggets and French fries. Still others may not consume enough calories, or they may overdo it. And an alarming number eat sugary candy and fried foods, more than is good for playing sports or for the growing body.

According to a 2011 review study from the University of Minnesota, sports-playing children (6 to 12 years of age) and teens (13 to 18 years of age) eat some of the worst diets on the planet, consuming more fast food, sugar-sweetened beverages, and calories.[1] On a positive note, the same study showed that young athletes eat more fruits, vegetables, and dairy products (a good thing) than their nonplaying counterparts.

Not only are the diets of young athletes loaded with nutrient-poor, high-calorie foods, but the nutrition quality of these foods may be inad-equate for playing a sport. In a study of teen soccer players, many athletes were under-fueled (they ate fewer calories than needed) and short on carbohydrates and other nutrients like folate, calcium, and vitamin D; some even showed signs of deficiencies in iron and vitamin D.[2] Another study showed that adolescent swimmers were eating more fat than needed, especially the unhealthy kind—saturated fat—and were falling short in recommended amounts of calcium and vitamin D, and in their daily intake of fruits, vegetables, grains, and dairy products.[3] These studies confirm what is already obvious in the world of youth sports: young athletes aren't fueling for performance. Instead, they may be creating nutritional deficits or excesses that rob them of their athletic potential.

Ironically, we live in a world where athleticism and physical activity are equated with health and vitality. Some parents believe that keeping a child active is all it takes to prevent poor eating or weight problems. But this is not true. What many parents don't understand is that more training and possessing the latest performance gear aren't enough. Good nutrition is the secret for physical health and athletic ability, now and in the future.

Yes, nutrition is the most overlooked weapon in the arsenal parents can use as they encourage their kids to play youth sports. Whether you're a newbie sports parent looking to make sure your athlete eats well or a veteran parent who wants to eke out every possible advantage, optimal nutrition will make a difference. Get it right and you will reap the rewards of an energetic, focused, fueled athlete who is ready at game time. Get it wrong and you will have the opposite—a distracted, hungry, lethargic athlete who struggles through practices and competitions. A solid nutrition program has the power to launch your young athlete to the next level. By the same token, poor nutrition can keep him in a holding pattern or even worsen his health.

I can't promise you that a healthy diet will translate to a 100% improvement in your child's athletic capabilities (to date no research confirms this), but there is plenty of information that suggests that nutrition can make a significant impact on your athlete's performance. The foods and beverages athletes eat can beef them up or lean them out, energize them or slow them down, keep them going or cause them to waver midway through a workout, or even keep them playing instead of being benched due to illness. When thoughtfully planned, the foods we feed our athletes, and how we feed them, can fuel them to the next level of success.

"You've changed the entire way I think about nutrition, and the way I feed my athlete," said Liza, mom of 14-year-old rower Drew, who was striving to find the right balance of food and calories. "I don't even think about food the same way." Liza's new understanding of sports nutrition changed everything for her and her son, helping to improve his weight, health and performance. And this is exactly what I intend to do for you— change the way you think about and execute food and the task of feeding your young athlete.

Nutrition and the Young Athlete

While participation in youth sports is growing by leaps and bounds, good nutrition is too often sidelined by a lack of proper sports nutrition guidance for young athletes, including a lack of age-appropriate information, inappropriate food offerings on the field, poor eating habits, the time limitations of busy parents, and much more. It's not easy to pull out your secret weapon—solid nutrition—and gain the edge in competition. To deliver good nutrition in today's sports world, you have to jump through a lot of hoops. And that requires understanding what's going on in youth sports. Let's take a look at some of the issues.

Increasing Participation

Youth sports are exploding in popularity, and organized sports continue to gain traction. According to a report titled, "Go Out and Play: Participation in Team or Organized Sports," prepared by the Women's Sports Foundation, 69% of girls and 75% of boys participate in organized or team sports annually.[4] The National Federation of State High School Associations (NFHS) found that some 7.7 million high school students played a sport during the 2012–2013 school year.[5] And about 46.5 million children play sports each year, with children 13 to 14 years old driving the biggest increases in sports participation, according to a survey by the National Sporting Goods Association.[6]

That's a mind-boggling number of young people who are active in sports. Some of these athletes play recreational sports, participating each week in one to three nights of practice and one or two games. Others are more serious, even elite, athletes who practice most days of the week (sometimes twice daily) and compete more than once a week. Without quality nutrition and the right approach, these athletes risk lackluster performance, nutrient deficiencies, and growth disturbances, as well as a lifetime of bad eating habits.

Missing the Boat

Many parents will pay almost anything to improve their child's athletic skills, according to Mark Hyman in his book, *The Most Expensive Game in Town: The Rising Cost of Youth Sports and the Toll on Today's Families*.[7] He estimates that parents spend thousands of dollars every year to keep their children involved and competitive in sports, footing the bill for camps, club sports, travel, and equipment, even in the face of financial strain. Ironically, parents miss the boat on one of the easiest and most obvious advantages available to them—good nutrition. Powerful, proven, and performance-enhancing, the right nutrition increases the competitive ability and athleticism of just about any athlete.

While we perceive playing sports as a healthy endeavor, it doesn't guarantee that your child will actually *be* healthy. Some of the latest information about youth sports suggests that athletes are not automatically becoming healthier because they play sports, in fact, they may be faced with a greater risk of childhood obesity.[8] Parents who try to feed their athletes well wrestle with a host of nutrition-related issues: the temptation to eat junk food, food marketing targeted at kids and teens, time pressures, and the normal social-emotional developmental changes that ebb and flow with childhood. The bottom line: it's not easy to raise a healthy athlete.

Another concern is the potential energy demand of sports during a time when young athletes are growing and developing. As athletes crank out grueling workouts, their bodies are tapping into available energy and nutrients for growth. This sets up a unique, once-in-a-lifetime situation for growing athletes. Not only do they need to eat to compete; they also need to eat to grow. If you don't know how to nourish and feed your athlete for growth and sport, you may find that nutrition is your enemy. Poor nutrition can actually work *against* your best intentions and your child's health and performance.

Barriers to Healthy Nutrition for Your Athlete

The youth sports nutrition world has never been more confusing. One coach advocates a no-sugar diet, while another routinely sips on a Big Gulp soda. One family deals with a crazy sports schedule by routinely visiting the drive-through or calling their favorite take-out joint, while another family devotedly packs up the cooler or turns on the slow cooker. Some athletes take performance aids (supplements), while others guzzle coffee. Even professional athletes smile for the camera, holding a triple-thick Oreo cookie. And let's not ignore the food that litters the fields, courts, and arenas of America's youth sporting venues. The ideal diet is at odds with the reality of the food landscape. Many barriers get in the way of good nutrition for our young athletes. Let's take a closer look at a few:

Nutrition Knowledge. Today's parents are more underprepared for nutrition and the job of feeding their kids than ever before. Fewer than 25% of parents know what foods to feed their kids, and 28% of adults don't know how to cook.[9,10] Even worse, only 77% of parents feel they can limit their kids' exposure to the junk foods and sweets that tempt them every day.[11] When it comes to sports nutrition, parents patch together information from books, magazines, and websites, but misinformation abounds, including what foods and fluids to give kids who play sports.[12] And when parents do seek out and find information on nutrition, it's more often than not based on recommendations for adult athletes. Using adult nutrition approaches for children and teens can have dangerous consequences, such as those seen with the consumption of energy drinks, which may cause caffeine toxicity, or pushing too much protein, which may cause dehydration and injure the kidneys. All told, parents are often under-informed or misguided when it comes to nutrition for their athletes.

Eating Habits. According to the 2015 Dietary Guidelines for Americans (DGA), many kids and teens have poor diets. Up to twenty-six percent of what kids and teens eat comes from sugary or salty snack foods, while important nutrients like calcium, folate, vitamins D, E, A, and C, magnesium, potassium, and fiber are crowded out of the diet, resulting in deficits.[13] The risk for teens increases as their nutrient requirements shoot up with their growth spurt and the potential unfolds for skipping meals, dieting, or snacking too much. Teens aged 14 to 18 eat the most sugar (up to 34 teaspoons [170 g] a day), and 92% of them snack, but not on the right foods.[14,15] Athletes aren't immune to these poor eating habits and food choices; many are missing out on sources of energy and important nutrients for performance, or overdoing it with too many calories, sugar, and fat. And depending on the sport, young athletes may be at risk for disordered eating or a full-blown eating disorder.

Inappropriate Food. Young athletes aren't any better than other kids— they may even be worse—at indulging in the unhealthy food that's front and center at competitions, in the school cafeteria, and in stores and food courts. Whether it is a gigantic double-chocolate-chip muffin or a high-protein energy bar, the truth is that it's not easy to eat "right" outside of the home. Even if healthy food is available, it's often served alongside candy and sweets. One of the biggest challenges is that sporting venues do little to promote the food athletes should be eating, making the healthy choice the hard choice.

Time Crunch. Work schedules and the crush of activities outside the office and workplace—including practices and games on weeknights and weekends—can lead to stress for parents at mealtime. Making things worse is the fact that many moms and dads have limited cooking skills. To make life easier, families may resort to fast food, take-out, or packaged meals and snacks, which can tip the balance of eating to the unhealthy side.

Persuasive Media. Young athletes are uniquely susceptible to adopting unhealthy behaviors like eating junk food, using performance-enhancing aids, and dieting. The pressure comes from peers, the media, and even professional athletes. Athletes are also lured by the muscular, fit ideal of the athletic body portrayed in magazines and on the Internet and TV. These body "ideals" are hard to come by, especially when you're young and growing or genetically inclined to be bigger or smaller, and may prove problematic to self-esteem and the development of good eating habits.

Nutrition Attitude. You can eat anything and then burn it off exercising— or so the popular myth promises. The young athlete is likely to develop this "eat anything" attitude toward food and nutrition unless parents have a handle on the purpose of food as fuel for exercise. The truth is, the eating patterns of the young athlete become the eating habits of the adult. If kids and teens are loading up on fatty, high-calorie, sugary foods now, they are more likely to do the same as adults, or at least have difficulty controlling their eating of such foods. Childhood habits are hard to break, and excess weight may become a harsh adult reality for the young athlete who has adopted the "eat anything and everything" attitude.

These barriers can make it difficult to feed your athlete a well-balanced, healthy diet tailored to fuel his or her athletic endeavors. Of course, it doesn't have to be this way. While you may feel overwhelmed by the obstacles you face, the right information and strategies can help you raise a healthy, strong, competitive athlete. You just need a reliable resource that lays out the research, translates it into everyday terms, and keeps you and your athlete motivated to be at the top of your nutrition game.

Why You Need *Eat Like a Champion*

It's not hard for an athlete to get off-track with nutrition. Part of the issue is that parents and coaches narrowly focus on the sport itself and the training that goes along with it, and give little attention to nutrition. The other problem is a lack of sports nutrition resources for the growing child and teen athlete. Until now, that is.

No earlier book has put all the youth sports nutrition information together: current research on young athletes, including factors related to their growth and development; practical strategies for daily eating; and ways to deal with specific nutrition challenges. This is what has been missing in youth sports—a "go to" resource that answers your questions, provides reliable guidance, addresses conflicting information about sports nutrition, and motivates everyone involved with young athletes to do their best with nutrition.

Eat Like a Champion makes the job of fueling top-notch athletes and helping them grow a lot easier.

Why I Wrote This Book

I'm a Hoosier (from Indiana), transplanted after college to the East Coast, where I started my career as a registered dietitian/nutritionist and raised my family. When I was young, my father wanted me and my siblings to play basketball (we lived in the land of Larry Bird and basketball, after all). I started in fifth grade and stuck with it through my junior year of high school. In the late 1970s and early 1980s, there wasn't much talk about sports nutrition. In fact, I don't remember taking even a water bottle to my 2-hour daily practice after school. I do remember the water fountain, though, and being super-hungry when I got home. The idea of an after-school snack to prepare me for exercise wasn't considered, nor was a recovery snack. What to eat for competition, hydration guidelines, and anything else related to nutrition and sport were not priorities for my parents, my coach, or me.

Sports trained me in the good habit of moving my body nearly every day. Unfortunately, because I was not fueling properly, I was often over-hungry when I got home, and I devoured whatever was in the cabinets, refrigerator, and pantry before dinner was even served. Looking back, I am certain I overate, although to look at me at the time, you wouldn't have known it. Those eating patterns that I developed as an athlete took a long time to correct.

Decades later, I am a mom with four active kids, two of whom are fairly serious about their sports. Even though I'm a dietitian and nutritionist, my nutrition and feeding efforts have occasionally come up short. In the midst of my daughter's growth spurt at age 13, I was certain she was becoming anemic. Training hard at swimming and growing like a weed, she became pale, fatigued, and obviously thinner, and she couldn't shake the bronchitis she had been battling for weeks. Off we went to the doctor, who ran tests. My daughter was slightly low on iron, so I had the job of getting her levels back up in a month or we would start iron supplementation. I bumped up the iron foods in our meals, added a vitamin C source to help her better absorb the iron, and began to fix her a nightly smoothie packed with fruits and spinach. Thankfully, she got better, and her iron status normalized.

You may wonder how a scenario like this could happen when I was an expert in the field of kids' nutrition, a professional who had worked with young athletes for many years. It happened for several reasons: I was juggling a private practice and writing my first book, *Fearless Feeding: How to Raise Healthy Eaters from High Chair to High School*, and my time for cooking and shopping was at an all-time low. My daughter was growing at an insane pace; she was not eating as well as I had thought at school; and she had increased her level of training as a senior swimmer. All these factors offset what was typically a well-run nutrition and feeding routine in our home. I credit my nutrition knowledge for catching and correcting the situation early.

I tell you this because I know what you're up against. I know it isn't easy to get nutrition on the table at night or to serve breakfast and pack lunches before 6 a.m. when you're juggling a full life. I know what it's like to make a healthy meal and have your athlete pick at it or refuse to eat it. I know how confusing nutrition advice for kids in sports can be. And I too get frustrated with the tantalizing concession stands and junk foods that seem to be there every time we turn around. It's all challenging for me, so I know it's probably challenging for you too.

That's why I wrote this book: to show you how to be successful with nutrition for your athlete, so that he or she can be successful in sports and develop the healthy eating habits that will pay big dividends over a lifetime. I explain nutrition science in parent-speak so you can understand the evidence and sift through the hype, keeping your athlete on a healthy course. I provide practical advice to get you through the day—from healthy snack ideas to getting dinner on the table when there is little time to cook. And I help you understand some of the most common challenges for young athletes, so you can step in when you need to. Everything you need to fuel a healthy, competitive athlete is right here—literally in your hands and at your fingertips.

What's in This Book

All the training in the world won't make up for poor nutrition. What your athlete needs is good nutrition served up regularly. And what you need is this book—a practical nutrition resource to guide you along the way, whether you're raising a recreational athlete or the next Tom Brady.

Part I of this book fills you in on the basics of nutrition, from specific sports and the calories they burn to growth needs and expectations for the child and teen athlete. Chapter 1 explains what to expect as your young athlete grows and develops. You'll understand how nutrition changes when growth starts to take off during puberty, and how that impacts your athlete's eating and his or her nutritional requirements. Chapter 2 discusses macronutrients (protein, carbohydrate, and fat), explains where to find them in food, and describes how much of each is needed for exercise. You will also understand the dangers of getting too much, and too little, of these nutrients. Chapter 3 is a primer on the micronutrients (vitamins and minerals), including how they function, how much kids and teens need, the critical ones for sport and growth, and common food sources. Chapter 4 discusses hydration, and explains how to determine your athlete's fluid needs and the best sources with which to hydrate, including a few yummy recipes.

Part II takes the research outlined in Part I and makes it practical. Chapter 5 shows you how to balance meals and get them on the table quickly, and lays out resources to use for fast at-home meals. And I address the latest research on the benefits of family meals, showcasing how and why you should get your athlete seated at the dinner table as many evenings as possible. I also discuss what to order when you are eating out. Chapter 6 covers snacking, both before and after exercise, describes healthy homemade snacks (along with a few recipes), and explains how to choose a packaged snack. Nutrient timing (when athletes eat) is a big deal in sports nutrition; I help you understand the benefits and provide the latest guidelines. Chapter 7 ends Part II with the lowdown on supplements, performance enhancers, and energy drinks, including the dangers of using them with children and teens, and findings from the most recent research.

Part III addresses the hurdles young athletes face, from managing weight to dieting and the food environment surrounding sports. Chapter 8 discusses healing the athlete's body using food, and I cover injury, chronic medical conditions, and eating disorders. Chapter 9 digs into special diets for young athletes, and has a special section on the vegetarian athlete. Chapter 10 ends the book with advice on changing the culture of sports nutrition on athletic fields, arenas, and courts. Included are tools to improve the food landscape, including a sample note to parents about snacks and healthy concession-stand items.

Communicating sports nutrition science isn't always easy, and some pages are filled with numbers, common values, and metrics, especially in Part I. If you're not a numbers person or if you have a new athlete, you can ignore these numbers, as you will still get the big picture. They're here because I am frequently asked for the details, especially by the parents of athletes who are high-level competitors. While this information may be a little "heady," glossing over or simplifying it won't help you in the long run, particularly if your athlete continues in sports. You'll also read case studies throughout the book, inspired by real athletes and families. These stories help bring sports nutrition for young athletes—its challenges and solutions—alive.

I want you to understand why recommendations for youth sports nutrition are what they are. You need to have a resource on hand now, when your little athlete is bombarded with junk food on the soccer field and you are simply trying to survive dinner, and in the future, when your teen wants to be a vegan, try a supplement, or wants to lose weight—or better yet, excel in sports beyond your imagination.

Notes

1. Nelson TF, Stovitz S, Thomas M, LaVoi N, Bauer K, Neumark-Sztainer D. "Do youth sports prevent pediatric obesity? A systematic review and commentary." *Curr Sports Med Rep.* 10 (2011): 360–370.
2. Gibson JC, Stuart-Hill L, Martin S, Gaul C. "Nutrition status of junior elite Canadian female soccer athletes." *Int J Sport Nutr Exerc Metab.* 21 (2011): 507–514.
3. Collins A, Ward K, Mirza B, Slawson D, McClanahan B and Vukadinovich C. "Comparison of nutritional intake in US adolescent swimmers and non-athletes." *Health.* 4 (2012): 873–880.
4. "Go Out and Play: Participation in Team or Organized Sports." Women's Sports Foundation. http://www.womenssportsfoundation.org/home/research/articles-and-reports/mental-and-physical-health/go-out-and-play.
5. "2012–2013 High School Athlete Participation Survey." National Federation of State High School Associations. http://www.nfhs.org/Participation Statics/PDF/2013-14%20NFHS%20Handbook_pgs52-70.pdf.
6. "Sports Participation in 2010 Survey." National Sporting Goods Association. http://www.nsga.org/i4a/pages/index.cfm?pageID=4492.
7. Hyman M. *The Most Expensive Game in Town: The Rising Cost of Youth Sports and the Toll on Today's Families.* Boston: Beacon Press, 2012.
8. Nelson, op. cit.

9. Moag-Stahlberg A. "The state of family nutrition and physical activity: Are we making progress?" American Dietetic Association. http://www.eatright .org/foundation/fnpa/.

10. "What's keeping Americans out of their kitchens? National survey reveals the top excuses for not cooking." Bosch Appliance. http://www.bosch-home .com/us/about-bosch/press-room/press-releases/press-releases-detail .html?pressrelease=what-s-keeping-americans-out-of-their-kitchens -national-survey-reveals-the-top-excuses-for-not-cooking~12154.

11. "Parents concerned, but confused about how to fix childhood obesity." Mintel. http://www.mintel.com/press-centre/food-and-drink/parents-concerned -but-confused-about-how-to-fix-childhood-obesity.

12. Barton Straus L. "Survey shows parents confusion on nutrition." http:// www.momsteam.com/nutrition/survey-shows-parent-confusion-on -nutrition.

13. U.S. Department of Agriculture and U.S. Department of Health and Human Services. "*Dietary Guidelines for Americans, 2015.*" Available at: http://www.health.gov/dietaryguidelines/2015-scientific-report/PDFs/ Scientific-Report-of-the-2015-Dietary-Guidelines-Advisory-Committee. pdf.

14. Reedy J, and Krebs-Smith SM. "Dietary sources of energy, solid fats, and added sugars among children and adolescents in the United States." *J Am Diet Assoc.* 110 (2010): 1477–1484.

15. Sebastian RS, Goldman JD, and Enns CW. "Snacking patterns of US adolescents. What we eat in America. NHANES 2005–2006." *Food Surveys Research Group. Dietary Data Brief, No. 2* (2010).

PART I

Nutrition Rules and Regulations

CHAPTER 1

The Growing Athlete: Body and Brain

What the mind of man can conceive and believe, it can achieve.
—Napoleon Hill, personal success author

Linda was the mom of twin girls who were volleyball players. At 14, they were playing on a new club team with other girls aged 15, 16, and 17. When Linda looked at the 10 members of the team lined up side by side, she noticed how thin her girls appeared. "My girls look like sticks compared to the other girls on the team!" she said. "I'm going to sign them up for some personal training so they'll beef up."

Whoa. Wait a minute. Linda didn't understand how varied body shapes and sizes are during puberty. In fact, if you lined up 10 girls or boys in this age range, you would see what Linda saw: a wide variety of body shapes and sizes. Puberty is the period of life when growth is rapid and individuality is the name of the game. Linda's girls hadn't filled out yet, though they were as tall as most of their teammates. I knew they were going to grow more and gain weight over the next couple of years simply because of their age. And no amount of personal training would accelerate this process.

From the ages of 8 to 18, children change dramatically. Children of ages 6 to 12 years are often sticklike figures, with barely any muscles, who gradually develop into busty, hippy girls and muscle-popping, hairy, almost-men boys through adolescence (13 to 18 years) and the process of puberty. It's during this 10-year phase that the most apparent physical changes in young athletes occur, markedly altering their physical presence and abilities. Naturally, this growth period, especially puberty, has a steep energy demand—hence the voracious appetite that often develops during this time.

Adding sports to the mix increases the overall calorie cost for the growing athlete. Depending on the nature of the sport, that cost will vary. For example, a rower will burn more calories in an hour than will a baseball player. It's important to know how many calories the various sports burn as you begin to understand your athlete's appetite and shape his or her approach to eating.

There's also a lot going on inside a young person's mind—hopes, fears, desires, and social pressures. Paying attention to your athlete's social-emotional development, or what's happening below the surface, will help you understand the motivations behind the food choices and eating behaviors you see.

In this chapter, I will explain critical aspects of a typical young athlete's overall body growth—in particular the muscles and bones—as well as how social and emotional developmental changes affect nutrition and eating. Let's get started so you have a basis and understanding for meeting the energy needs of your athlete.

Growing for the Gold

Parents of sports-playing kids are often caught up in the moment, carting them to and from practices and games and watching them play. Many parents juggle meals and snacks along with the demands of their jobs, carpooling, and running the house, and meet the demands of hunger on the fly.

I've heard countless complaints from parents about their child's poor eating habits. I've seen many a young athlete eat Skittles during a competition, load up on donuts before a tournament, and recover from an intensive workout with pizza, dessert, and other unhealthy options.

However, as much as kids and teens would like to use Olympic swimmer Michael Phelps's approach to eating—endless amounts of high-calorie food such as hamburgers, pizza, and sweets—the truth is they really can't. Most young athletes have nowhere near Phelps's athletic abilities and training schedule, and therefore cannot burn off the vast number of calories that go along with his eating patterns.

Physical growth is a progressive endeavor. Until young athletes reach their adult size, shape, and weight, they will be growing and changing, affecting their energy and nutrient needs.

Before puberty sets in, boys and girls grow at a steady rate and are similar in their body composition (muscle and body fat balance) and nutritional requirements.[1] As puberty begins, around age 10 to 11 years for girls and 2 years later for boys, the energy requirements for normal growth and development escalate. If athletes eat poorly, they may experience nutritional deficiencies that can impact not only their athletic performance, but also their overall growth and physical development, as well as their abilities to succeed academically.[2] Chronic under-eating may lead to short stature, delayed puberty, irregular menstrual periods for girls, poor bone health, and a higher risk of injuries.

Table 1-1 details the annual growth expectations for kids and teens aged 8 to 18 along with their energy needs, expressed in numbers of calories, when they engage in varying levels of physical activity.[3,4]

As mentioned above, up to about age 10, kids grow at a steady pace, with occasional spurts and lags in growth. Using the body mass index (BMI) chart, a growth chart that details overall weight and height progression, will help you evaluate your athlete's growth. You can calculate the BMI at http://nccd.cdc.gov/dnpabmi/Calculator.aspx, or simply check in with your doctor. You'll want to see steady and consistent increments in overall growth year after year; any significant change—up or down—on the growth and BMI curves should be cause for further investigation with your pediatrician.

The BMI compares an absolute weight status in relation to an individual's height. Once calculated, BMI values are classified as normal, overweight, obese, or underweight. In athletes, BMI is a tricky tool to use, as

Table 1-1 Average Energy Needs and Annual Growth

Age	Energy Needs: Sedentary (Calories/Day)	Energy Needs: Moderately Active (Calories/Day)	Energy Needs: Active (Calories/Day)	Average Weight Gain	Average Height Gain
8 years	Female: 1,200–1,400	1,400–1,600	1,400–1,800	4–5 lb per year	2–2.5 inches (in) per year
	Male: 1,200–1,400	1,400–1,600	1,600–2,000	4–5 lb per year	2–2.5 in per year
9 to 13 years	Female: 1,400–1,600	1,600–2,000	1,800–2,200	5–7 lb per year; a 10-year-old may gain up to 9 lb per year	2.5 in per year; varies with onset of puberty
	Male: 1,600–2,000	1,800–2,200	2,000–2,600	A 10-year-old may gain up to 9 lb per year	2.5 in per year; varies with onset of puberty
14 to 18 years	Female: 1,800	2,000	2,400	Average weight gain is 21 lb during adolescence	Maximal height growth is 3.3–3.5 in per year; almost 10 in gained during puberty
	Male: 2,000–2,400	2,400–2,800	2,800–3,200	Average weight gain is 34 lb during adolescence	Maximal height growth is 3.7–4.1 in per year; almost 11 in gained during puberty

it may reflect a high muscle mass when measuring total body weight. Since athletes tend to have more muscle, especially teens, and muscle weighs more than fat, the athlete may be incorrectly identified as overweight or obese. A good example of this is the husky football player—if his BMI were measured, it may be on the higher side, even indicating overweight or obesity, yet he could be sporting minimal body fat, and lots of muscle. It's important to keep this in mind when using weight measures. The ideal use of the BMI is as a tracking tool, so you can note any deviations from your athlete's normal growth pattern.

It's normal to see peaks and valleys in appetite, as this relates to what's happening with growth. You may see more hunger during growth spurts and low or normal appetite during slowed growth. It's also completely normal for an athlete to be extra hungry after a sports practice and not as hungry during days off.

Table 1-1 lays out the expectations and general population averages of appropriate height and weight gains for kids between the ages of 8 and 18. These averages should be used as reference points for deciding what is normal, and what isn't, when it comes to your athlete's growth. That growth will reflect children's genetic makeup, the quantity and quality of the food they eat, and the balance between their nutritional intake and the demands of both physical development and the exercise they undertake.

Also critical to normal growth and development is sleep—the time when the body restores and heals itself following the activities of the day. According to the National Sleep Foundation, your younger child should be getting about 9 to 11 hours of sleep per night and your teen at least 8 hours. Getting teenagers to catch that many zzz's is a challenge, as their circadian biological clock makes them alert later at night, making it difficult for them to fall asleep before 11 p.m.[5]

What does this all mean? It means you can do a lot to optimize growth, like feeding your athlete healthy food most of the time and making sure he or she is getting enough sleep. However, you can't change what nature intended. Your naturally short-statured son isn't likely to experience a surge in height and become the center on the basketball team, and your slight-bodied track athlete daughter may struggle with being thin. And no matter how hard you try to get your older athlete to sleep, you just might have to settle for weekends of sleeping in.

Where Do All the Calories Go?

Have you ever wondered how calories are dispersed throughout the body? A large number go to what experts call resting energy expenditure (REE), which represents about 50% of our caloric needs. Our bodies are actually hard at work while we sleep, burning calories by pumping blood, working our lungs while we breathe, making new tissue, and repairing any damage to muscles that has occurred from exercise. The

REE ranges from 1,000 to 1,500 calories, depending on factors like weight, height, age, sex, and race. When we are awake, we need the other 50% of our calories to provide energy for our movement, thinking, and normal activity. Remember, those total calorie needs are highly variable between individuals. What's unique to children and teens is that, pound for pound, their bodies require more calories than adults because of the added demand of growth.

Appetite

For most athletes, their natural appetite will drive food intake and growth. Letting appetite take charge is the best bet for getting an accurate sense of how many calories they need. As the internal regulator of food intake, an athlete's appetite relies on hormones like ghrelin, which triggers hunger, and leptin, which shuts it off. However, the regulation of appetite isn't a simple matter because hormones are complicated, and they aren't the only things that influence appetite. Other factors—including, of course, the appearance and taste of food—can make young athletes want to eat even when they're not physically hungry.

Kids and teens don't always eat based on a good sense of their appetite. We only have to look to the obesity statistics to see that there is a problem. One in three children and teens is overweight or obese. Part of this problem is due to what and how much they eat. Twenty-percent of kids' daily calories come from snacks, and 34 teaspoons (136 g) of sugar are consumed by typical teens each day.[6,7] Eating hefty snacks and excessive sugar often translates to overeating. Additionally, some kids eat without thinking, not paying attention to or caring about what or how much they've eaten. They may eat mindlessly or with an "absence of hunger," a term coined by researchers in the obesity field that means eating for reasons other than hunger—like boredom, celebration, or sadness—which has been linked to overeating and weight gain. Other kids eat because something looks yummy or tastes good, with little thought of what the food contains. This, by itself, isn't necessarily a problem, but kids and teens do it far too often.

It's important that your athlete recognize physical hunger. If he is out of touch with this, he may not know when to eat, when to stop, or how much to eat. As a result, he may fail to tame what I call "head hunger"—other reasons for eating that aren't related to nourishment. You can help your athlete differentiate head hunger ("That looks so good, I want to eat it" or "I just want some crunchy, fatty, salty, sweet junk food") from physical hunger (tummy growling, headache, moodiness, and other symptoms of low blood sugar) by offering an apple or a sandwich when he says he's hungry. If he'd rather have ice cream, he's probably got head hunger. Appetite isn't the only thing that drives eating and growth, other factors play a role.

Puberty

Everything you thought you knew about kids and nutrition changes once puberty begins. As mentioned earlier, most girls enter puberty between the ages of 10 and 11; boys begin the process about 2 years later, between the ages of 12 and 13.[8] During puberty, lots of changes happen, including height growth, weight gain, bone lengthening, muscle growth, and, for girls, menstruation.

When the puberty hormones estrogen (for girls) and testosterone (for boys) start to rev up in the body, physical changes begin. The little fat roll that forms around girls' bellies at ages 10 and 11 (or even a little bit earlier) is a normal part of getting ready for menstruation. These fat stores produce estrogen, the hormone responsible for regular periods. Girls who form this belly early will be more likely to start their periods earlier than girls who develop this pudginess later. Girls' bellies will gradually disappear as their breasts develop and their hips widen.

Too much exercise, or under-eating, can disrupt or delay the start of menstruation, especially in girls who are at the elite level of their sport. The intensity and duration of exercise—and the calorie burn—can lead to low body-fat stores and thus a suppression of estrogen. Studies have detailed this effect in gymnasts, dancers, swimmers, runners, and participants in other high-calorie-burning, appearance-focused sports. However, young girls or teens who exercise less than 15 hours per week do not tend to show disruption in menstruation or delays in sexual maturation.[9]

The menstrual cycle increases the need for iron in all girls. Unfortunately, some aren't getting enough iron in their diets, which contributes to iron deficiency, or anemia, which is problematic for any girl, but especially for the serious athlete.[10] A nonathlete who is iron deficient or anemic may experience symptoms such as pale skin, weakness, shortness of breath, fatigue, frequent illnesses or infections, and dizziness. Any young athlete with an iron deficiency will likely experience the same symptoms, but additionally see negative effects on athletic performance such as early fatigue and reduced stamina. Be sure to read Chapter 3 for more details on iron deficiency and the foods that are good sources of iron.

The key hormone for boys is testosterone, a natural steroid hormone (meaning it is produced by the body). It is often referred to as the "sex hormone," and promotes muscle growth during puberty. When levels of testosterone peak (around 14 to 16 years of age), muscles start to bulk up. The precise timing of the testosterone peak varies from individual to individual and is mostly related to heredity. The other signs of puberty in boys include stinky armpits; pimples; hair growth on the face, armpits, and other areas; and voice changes. While not bulky yet, muscles for both girls and boys get stronger with exercise, which is something to celebrate and watch for in athletic performance.

Muscles

Muscles develop, in part, based on hormone concentrations of testosterone in both males and females. Males have higher circulating levels of testosterone; their muscles eventually get bigger and bulkier than female's muscles. And, no, you cannot do anything (safely or legally) to make them pop out earlier. Although muscles start to become defined in the early teens, fat-free mass (muscle and bone) typically reaches maturity around age 19 or 20 in males; in young female athletes, it's earlier, between 15 and 16.[11] Eventually males will have more muscle—and, in turn, more strength and speed—than girls, who carry more fat.

Common sense suggests, and research proves, that more muscle translates to positive performance outcomes, while too much body fat negatively impacts performance, especially in movement sports like running, vaulting, and jumping.[12] Many elements go into muscle development and performance, but the playing field is not level when it comes to body composition. It's a good thing boys compete against boys, and girls against girls.

According to a 2010 report published in *Pediatrics*, the ability of young people to gain muscular strength increases with age and maturity.[13] Yet children can benefit at any age from strength training, which conditions the nervous system and muscles to interact more efficiently, resulting in increased strength. Researchers believe the best time to start strength training is between 7 and 12 years of age because at that point the nervous system is very plastic and receptive. Consistency in repeated sessions yields the most strength.

This is music to many parents' and coaches' ears, but remember that kids participating in resistance training need supervision to prevent injuries. According to the Center for Injury Research and Policy at Nationwide Children's Hospital, young people 13 to 24 years of age sustained the highest rate of weight-training–related injuries, and 90% of the injuries were related to the use of free weights.[14] Instead of using free weights, your athlete should use his or her own body weight—it's readily available and less likely to cause injury.

Resistance training (pull-ups, push-ups, planks, sit-ups, and even carrying the groceries and shoveling snow) helps young muscles get stronger, which may improve athleticism. Teen athletes have to work their muscles if they want them to become bigger, bulkier, and more defined. Food alone, or loading up on protein supplements, won't bulk up muscles. If athletes don't exercise their muscles and keep their bodies in caloric balance, that extra protein can turn into extra calories and take the form of body fat, which can slow any athlete down. I'll cover this in more detail in Chapter 2.

Bones

I want to stress the importance of bone growth during childhood. As one of the most obvious changes during the growing years, bones get longer (hence the amazing increases in height) and thicken until the early 20s, when they finish growing. Adequate amounts of dietary calcium and other nutrients like vitamin D are essential not only for building bones during childhood, but also for retaining bone density into late adulthood. Exercise and resistance training help this growth process by producing denser bone tissue and thus stronger bones, which can mean fewer bone problems, like osteoporosis (porous, weak bones with higher fracture risk), later in life.

Certain sports—gymnastics, hurdling, judo, karate, volleyball, and other jumping sports—increase bone mineral density. High-intensity sports, like sprint running, have also been shown to have a positive effect on bone. Nonimpact sports like swimming, cycling, and sailing are not associated with improvements in bone structure. Swimmers tend to have lower bone density in their legs, partly due to the low impact involved in swimming.[15] If your athlete plays a nonimpact sport, you might want to add a component of resistance training or a high-impact or high-intensity sport to his or her training profile to promote bone health.

Exercise and growth—both important factors in achieving success in any sports activity—require calories. When overall calories are insufficient, your athlete may experience problems with growth, including short stature and late onset of puberty, as well as low energy and fatigue. I'll get picky about which foods are the best calorie sources in Chapter 5, because the foods athletes eat do matter, despite what you may see them eating in ads on TV or in magazines.

Matching Calories for Growth and Sport

One burning question for many parents and coaches of young athletes is *"How many calories does my athlete need?"* While you won't find a lot of research about calorie requirements for young athletes, it's known that children are less efficient with calorie burning during exercise than are adults. As such, they need more calories per pound compared to adults, who are more metabolically efficient.[16] One reason for this difference in calorie requirements is that children have shorter limbs than adults, so when they run they use more steps to cover the same distance as an adult, resulting in more energy expenditure in comparison. Another factor is that children use different energy sources for exercise, particularly fat over carbohydrate, something I will cover later. This difference in energy sourcing enhances their ability to sustain aerobic exercise (endurance-based exercise like running, biking, skiing, swimming, basketball, and soccer), but reduces their capacity for anaerobic exercise (high-intensity, short-term activity like short sprints, relays, weight lifting, baseball, kickball).

This fact helps explain why children can run and run and never seem to get tired. As children get older, their sourcing of energy changes to that of an adult (using carbohydrate over fat as an energy source), as does their metabolic efficiency with exercise.[17]

The estimated energy requirements shown in Table 1-1 take into account resting energy expenditure, physical activity, and growth requirements for daily energy needs. Most young athletes would be categorized as *active* or *very active*.

For the teen athlete who is exercising for longer than 2 hours at a time, here's a general rule of thumb for estimating daily calorie requirements:

Girls: 20 to 23 calories per pound of body weight (44–51 cals/kg)

Boys: 20 to 26 calories per pound of body weight (44–57 cals/kg)

Energy needs will go up when the duration of exercise is longer. Likewise, exercising for less than 2 hours means fewer calories burned, so shoot for fewer calories per pound (the lower end of the range above). The Academy of Nutrition and Dietetics recommends 3,000 to 4,000 calories per day for active males and 2,200 to 3,000 calories per day for active females.[18]

Yet another way to estimate the calorie burn of various sports is to look at the (limited amount of) research on young athletes in specific sports, which I have included in Table 1-2.[19] You won't find every sport listed here, nor will you find values for both sexes in some cases. This is because the research in youth sports is still emerging. If you're inclined to estimate the calories for your athlete, look at the different ways above and do an average of the results. Last, be careful using websites that offer such information, as it may be pulled from adult research, which may over- or underestimate calories for young athletes.

I wish I could give you a hard-and-fast rule for estimating calorie needs, but the truth is that calorie needs are highly variable from one athlete to another. The best way to determine your children's requirements is to allow them to lead with their appetite, offer plenty of nutritious food, understand the ballpark needs related to their normal growth and sport, and monitor their weight and growth.

In most sports, training sessions and practices offer more consistent exercise than a competition. Calorie-burning activities during training

Table 1-2 The Calorie Cost of Selected Sports for Young Athletes

Sport	Sex	Age (Years)	Calories
Swimming	Males	9–13	27 calories per pound
	Females	18–20	2,300–3,100 calories per day
Cross-country running	Females	18–22	2,300 ± 950 calories per day
Gymnastics	Females	7–10 11–14	1,650 ± 360 calories per day 1,700 ± 400 calories per day
Figure skating	Females	13–17	1,675 ± 700 calories per day
	Males	14–17	2,300–2,600 ± 900 calories per day
Wrestling	Males	15–17	2,700 ± 800 calories per day
Karate	Females	18–19	1,950 ± 400 calories per day
	Males	19–20	2,700 ± 700 calories per day
Ice hockey	Males	12	2,400 ± 500 calories per day
Football	Males	12–14 15–18	2,500 ± 900 calories per day 3,350 ± 1,600 calories per day
Volleyball	Females	14–19	1,600 ± 800 calories per day
Soccer	Males	15–19	3,950 ± 1,100 calories per day
Basketball	Females	19	2,000 ± 150 calories per day

typically include repetitive movements, running, or weight training. During competition, though, the calorie burn varies based on the sport. For example, a soccer or basketball game offers few breaks for resting, so the activity level is consistently elevated, whereas at a swim meet or rowing regatta there can be hours between races (which are short bursts of activity), allowing for plenty of downtime and energy conservation.

High and Low Calorie Burners

Sports differ when it comes to calorie burning. Some are high-calorie-burning sports and some are low burners. The intensity of individual aspects of an exercise can vary as well; for example, gymnastics can be a high-calorie-burning sport if the workout is tumbling.

High calorie burners: basketball, running/track, distance running, swimming, figure skating, ice hockey, soccer, rowing, elite-level tennis

Low calorie burners: baseball, football, gymnastics, martial arts, recreational tennis, wrestling

Keep in mind that each athlete has an individual response to exercise based on age, sex, pubertal stage, nutritional status, genetic makeup, physical prowess, and more.

Elite athletes tend to adapt to heavy training by resting. Athletes who intensively train for their sport may compensate by becoming more sedentary during the day, thus conserving their energy.[20] The elite lacrosse player who hangs out on the couch for hours after practice is an example of this phenomenon. This self-regulation of energy expenditure is a way for an athlete to stay in calorie balance.

When the Growing Gets Tough

Growth doesn't always go so well, and sometimes participation in a sport is the culprit. Some sports, such as competitive tennis, may disrupt your child's appetite and food intake, creating a gap between (low) calorie intake and (high) energy burn that results in weight loss or a lack of normal weight gain. Other sports, like baseball, may not burn many calories at all and the opposite can occur—unwanted weight gain.

Fortunately, sophisticated equations that incorporate your athlete's REE, age, sex, sport, time spent exercising, and metabolic equivalents (the energy spent doing an activity, on average) can quantify his or her energy burn.[21] These equations are too complicated for the purposes of this book—mostly because they offer highly individualized results; a sports nutritionist can detail this information for your young athlete.

Sadie, a 15-year-old softball player, was mortified to find she was gaining weight after her season was over, and cut her calories to 1,200 a day. In essence, she went from one end of the spectrum, eating like she was a football player, to the other end, eating barely anything at all. Neither of these approaches was favorable—one meant becoming too heavy and the other left her under-fueled. She needed to understand a few things about managing her weight as an athlete:

- *Food is fuel.* An athlete's body depends on it. Nutritious food, in the right proportions and just the right amount to keep the fuel tank full, is optimal. Too little may cause early exhaustion and poor performance.
- *There's a balance to strike.* Weight gain comes from too much food, eating the wrong type, or not enough exercise. Likewise, weight loss comes from too little food or too much exercise. If weight gain or loss is occurring, the balance is off-kilter.
- *Weight stability is the name of the game.* During an athletic season, neither weight gain nor weight loss is desirable. If an athlete needs to lose weight, he should do it in the off-season. If dropping pounds is absolutely necessary during the season, seek out a professional for guidance, so that the athletic endeavors and the health of the player don't suffer. You can find more information about weight management in Chapter 9.

My advice for Sadie was to keep her food portions reasonable (see Chapter 5 for specifics), have a snack only once a day, and limit desserts to two or three times a week. I also suggested she do a better job of staying fit by exercising daily during the off-season.

When under-eating becomes significant, it can affect a child's growth. This happened to Jessie, a 13-year-old competitive swimmer. She put in six daily practices of 2 hours each, and sometimes did doubles, swimming in the early-morning hours and coming back again at night. Ironically, on these double days, she ate less than normal because she would lose her appetite, which isn't unusual after intense exercise. The rush to get to school and the limited time she had for eating put Jessie in a difficult situation—a negative calorie balance. Rail thin and exhausted, she came to me for help.

Jessie and her family didn't fully understand the implications of the calorie cost of swimming, as well as her present stage of growth—the beginning of the adolescent growth surge; both were increasing her calorie needs. Once we quantified the needs of both her growth and her sport, it was easy to see that Jessie was way behind. To address the difference, I put her on a meal plan that started with a preload snack for early-morning practices that used Banana Pucks (see Chapter 6 for the recipe) or a handful each of nuts and dried fruit. I revamped her breakfast to include more calories and incorporate more fat—oatmeal made with whole milk, olive oil when cooking eggs, and avocado or nut butter in smoothies. We agreed on a lunch she could manage consistently, such as a meat and cheese sandwich with avocado or a peanut butter and jelly sandwich. I wanted Jessie to have a snack before her afternoon practice as well, something she could eat quickly on the way to the pool, like a granola bar, yogurt-covered raisins, or a few fig cookies. I also reviewed dinner options with her mom and dad, highlighting ways to pump up the calories such as sautéing veggies in oil or adding cheese or creamy salad dressing to salads. Finally, we added a bedtime snack—peanut butter toast, a bowl of cereal with milk, or a milkshake—to make sure calories were on board as she rested. Jessie's weight slowly increased, and she was better fueled for swimming.

You'll want to keep track of your young athlete's growth, which can be done at the pediatrician's office or at home with regular checks of her BMI. If you notice too much weight gain or signs of weight loss, help her get back on track. While you cannot force her to eat or reduce her intake, you can certainly set up an environment for success, which is what this book is all about. You'll find detailed advice on meals and snacks in Chapters 5 and 6.

Cracking the Brain Code

The young athlete's body isn't the only thing that's growing—although it's the most obvious change. Many changes are happening inside, particularly those involving the brain. Contending with grumpy, noncompliant teens who do whatever they want to do, rather than what you want them to do, is not easy for any parent. Watching your healthy eater at home turn into the cookie monster on the baseball field is no party either.

Many parents face the challenge and frustration of getting their young athletes to eat for sports, growth, and health. During this time, significant cognitive and social-emotional changes are afoot that influence how children and teens hear nutrition messages, determine which foods they choose to eat, and shape their motivation to prioritize nutrition. Knowing what's going on in your athlete's head helps you create positive motivation for eating well.

Cognitively Confused and Socially Motivated

There was no way 11-year-old Amy, a diver, was giving up her candy. She loved it too much. No matter how often she'd heard it was bad for her, she knew it tasted good, and that was all that mattered.

Children and teens, athletes or not, all travel through the same developmental phases related to their thinking and emotional growth. In the sports world, where children and teens experience early physical achievements, the brain marches to the beat of its own drum, cognitively speaking. Truth be told, even the most accomplished young athletes— including Olympians, no less—are still cognitively and emotionally "young." Although parents and other adults would like them to think and act older, the fact is that most kids and teens think and act according to their age.

Child psychologist Jean Piaget described children, ages 7 to 11 years, as black-and-white, right-or-wrong thinkers, limited in their abilities to see the long-term consequences of their actions.[22] This is why many children, like Amy, love junk foods—they taste good, are easy to get, and everyone (read: peers) is eating them. While coaches and parents can try to mold better eating habits, taste and popularity will mean more to your athlete than any logical argument that the junk is unhealthy.

So how do you handle this situation? Be the nutrition gatekeeper. Let in the food you approve, set limits and guidelines for eating candy and other junk food, and make healthy food look appealing and taste good. Setting policies such as "no candy during competition" or "healthy food only while training" can go a long way, as many children and preteen athletes are willing to follow rules and guidelines, especially when they are clear-cut.

The teenager is another animal to tame, however. While a teen's thinking becomes more complex, sensitive to others, and longer term in its perspective, the teen brain is also involved in what experts call a *remap-*

ping, or brain reorganization. In this multiyear process, unused neurons in the brain are pruned away, brain pathways are modified, and things "upstairs" are reorganized.[23] The process is comparable to an attic clean out. The brain saves the most important stuff, rearranges the storage bins (information), and throws away the garbage.

It's a well-accepted fact that the thinking and actions of teens don't always make sense. They behave in ways that are often impulsive, centered on reward (versus risk), and looking for a thrill. While teens can see consequences, they don't always think things through. The good news is that this remapping process runs its course by early adulthood, when the teen-turned-adult's thinking becomes even deeper, more forward thinking, and more insightful.

Cognitive changes can be challenging, but the social dynamics that younger kids and teens muddle through can also be real barriers to their health, wellness, and sports performance. According to child psychologist Erik Erikson, young children are peer-driven, learn everything under the sun (they're called "sponges" for a reason), and tend to listen to rules and defer to authority figures.[24] Meanwhile, their behavior, their successes and failures on and off the court, and feedback from the community influence the development of their self-esteem. When it comes to nutrition and food choices, if your child's friend is eating junk, then your little athlete will probably want to eat it too.

Teens are a little more complex in their social-emotional developmental progression, suggests Erikson. The young teen (between 13 and 15) is still influenced by peers and motivated to fit in, which makes him more susceptible to both peer and outside pressures. For example, if a popular Olympian is endorsing fast-food establishments, teen athletes may be keen on this food, ask for it, and eat it. As they grow older, by around age 17 or 18, their desire to be different emerges. This may lead to experimentation with diets, supplements, or other unhealthy behaviors. Some teens are more extreme in their pursuit of being different from others. Of course, every teen is an individual and will experience this stage of development in his or her own way.

Athleticism and playing a sport can have a great influence on the developing self-esteem of young people. Self-efficacy—believing in one's abilities—may stem from participating in athletics and increase self-esteem.[25] One study found higher academic scores and cognitive function in girl athletes, and lower depression and suicide rates in teens playing sports.[26] Finally, an athlete's fit appearance has been shown to elevate self-esteem.

Tips for Getting Your Young Athlete to Eat Well

While you want to help your young athlete achieve his or her best in the world of sports, food and eating are often areas where you may feel you're talking to a wall. Understanding your athlete's developmental stage and the secrets behind successful motivation will foster better communication. Here are a few tips:

- *Don't make your child or teen "different."* Children want to be the same—socially, in their appearance and accomplishments, emotionally, and yes, even with eating.
- *Move the mountain.* If you want your child or teen to snack on healthy foods, you'll have better luck if the whole team does it. Offer group snacks for the whole team, for instance, and your athlete will likely fall in step.
- *Keep it simple.* If you talk about nutrition and healthy eating, keep it basic and focus on aspects of the sport: strength, speed, endurance, and overall improvement. While you and I understand the long-term implications of nutrition on health and performance gains, younger kids don't really care, and teens won't until they are older.
- *Serve easy food.* Prepare healthy food, and make it easy to grab and go. Kids and teens will be more likely to eat food like fruit kabobs, mini-bagels and nut butter, or bagged trail mix that you prepare for them. Don't have sugary donuts, muffins, or candy around. Healthy food won't stand a chance.
- *Tap into pleasure.* Like exercising, eating healthy food can make young athletes *feel* healthy and energized. Eating junk can drag them down and make them feel heavy and lazy. Make sure you highlight these connections. The appearance, smell, and taste of food all are associated with the pleasure of eating well.

Motivation Moxie

One of the biggest challenges today's parents face is motivating their young athlete to *want* to eat well enough of the right foods, and in the right balance—for health and sport. "You don't really *create* motivation in your child," says Jonathan F. Katz, PhD, a clinical sports psychologist. "Kids need to internalize the importance of eating, sleeping, and training before they will be motivated to take care of their body for sport in a constructive way." Katz emphasizes that one of the most potent influences in young athletes' eating is what they see at home from their parents on a daily basis.

Modeling good eating behaviors every day makes the concept of healthy fueling for daily life a reality for your children. "Fueling for sport is simply an extension of what's eaten at home," Katz reminds us. "It's hard to get your kids to eat properly for competition and training if they're not doing it day to day."

Motivation is complex. While it involves many steps and theories, ultimately it's what leads to action. If your athlete is motivated to run faster, he or she will put every effort into doing so. Some kids may be motivated by a medal or by money, while others are satisfied knowing they've accomplished their goal, whether it's running faster, swimming longer, or nailing a routine without a mistake. What motivates your athlete may be a mystery to you, especially when it comes to eating well, but it doesn't have to be. Let's dig a little deeper.

Intrinsic (internal) motivation is lasting because it's a value system that resides within the individual, providing a compass and internal feedback on a young athlete's actions and behaviors. Experts in motivation have outlined three types of intrinsic motivation:

1. *Motivation to know*: doing something for the simple pleasure of learning—for example, watching a video on football plays to improve one's knowledge of strategy.
2. *Motivation to achieve*: doing something to surpass previous accomplishments, such as jumping a little bit farther in the long jump than the last time.
3. *Motivation to experience sensation*: doing something for appearances or sensory pleasure—trying a new food because it looks delicious

or getting the most valuable player award to add to the college application.

Extrinsic (external) motivation, like an award or money, hinges on receiving a reward unrelated to the activity. An example: a dollar for every second that runners take off their race time. Many athletes are motivated to push harder and perform better when there is a reward at the end.

Ultimately, though, the goal is to develop an appreciation for intrinsic reward, because this is what sticks. Intrinsic motivation leads to recurrent and sustained action. And external rewards, like ribbons or a few extra dollars, may not always be available. Molding an intrinsic motivation to eat well and improve is the real reward for all athletes, helping them along to excel in their sport and their life.

Laying the groundwork for your athletes' intrinsic motivation is your goal. You won't be able to "make" your children eat well (or practice, or sleep more, or any other desirable behavior), but if you behave strategically as you set up the food environment for success and model healthy eating from day to day, you will slowly help them along their developmental path and instill the ingredients for internal motivation.

Target the Nutrition Message

One aspect of motivating your athlete to eat well is to make sure nutrition messages are accurate and age-appropriate. Telling 8-year-old hockey enthusiasts that protein helps build muscle doesn't really motivate them to eat protein. ("What is protein, anyway?" they wonder.) On the other hand, explaining that "meat, milk, and beans are good for your muscles" is clearer and may motivate them to eat more of these foods.

Telling 14-year-old basketball-playing teens that they should load up on protein may result in excess protein consumption, which could be dehydrating or cause unwanted weight gain. Suggesting that they include a quality protein source like milk or cheese at each meal is more realistic and specific.

Make sure that the way you talk about nutrition and the messages you use are sensitive to what your young athlete *can* hear, not necessarily what you think he or she *should* hear.

Growth is one of the most fascinating things you will observe as your child morphs into a teen and then an adult. From physical changes to broader thinking patterns, all young athletes navigate the same waters—physically, cognitively, socially, and emotionally. Your job as captain of the ship is to stay on top of adequate food, nutrition, and growth while riding the rough waters of developmental changes and understanding your role in motivation—all without capsizing.

Notes

1. Rogol AD, Roemmich JN, and Clark PA. "Growth at puberty." *J Adolesc Health*. 31 (2002): 192–200.
2. Hoch AZ, Goossen K, and Kretschmer T. "Nutritional requirements of the child and teenage athlete." *Phys Med Rehabil Clin N Am*. 19 (2008): 373–398.
3. Rogol, op. cit.
4. U.S. Department of Agriculture and U.S. Department of Health and Human Services. "*Dietary Guidelines for Americans, 2015*." Available at: http://www .health.gov/dietaryguidelines/2015-scientific-report/PDFs/Scientific Report-of-the-2015-Dietary-Guidelines-Advisory-Committee.pdf.
5. "Children and Sleep." National Sleep Foundation. http://sleepfoundation org/sleep-topics/children-and-sleep.
6. "Child Obesity Facts." Centers for Disease Control and Prevention. http:// www.cdc.gov/healthyyouth/obesity/facts.htm.
7. Reedy J, and Krebs-Smith SM. "Dietary sources of energy, solid fats, and added sugars among children and adolescents in the United States." *J Am Diet Assoc*. 110 (2010): 1477–1484.
8. Rogol, op. cit., p. 196.
9. Meyer F, O'Connor H, and Shirreffs SM. "Nutrition for the young athlete." *J Sports Sci*. 25 (2007): S73–S82.
10. McManus AM, and Armstrong N, "Physiology of elite young female athletes." In: Medical Sports Science, ed. *The Elite Young Athlete*. Basel: S. Karger AG, 2011.
11. Ibid.
12. Malina RM, and Geithner CA. "Body composition of young athletes." *Am J Life Med*. 5 (2011): 262–278.
13. Behringer M, vom Heede A, Yue, Z, and Mester J. "Effects of resistance training in children and adolescents: a meta-analysis." *Pediatrics*. 126 (2010): e1190–e1210.

14. "New national study examines weight training-related injuries, Nationwide Children's." Newswise. http://www.newswise.com/articles/new-national -study-examines-weight-training-related-injuries.

15. Malina and Geithner, op. cit.

16. Georgopoulos NA, Roupas ND, Theodoropoulou A, Tsekouras A, Vagenakis AG, and Markou KE. "The influence of intensive physical training on growth and pubertal development in athletes." *Ann N Y Acad Sci*. 1205 (2010): 39–44.

17. Jeukendrup A and Cronin L. "Nutrition and elite young athletes," in The Elite Young Athlete. 56 (2011): 47–58. S Karger AG, Basel.

18. Rosenbloom C. "Teen nutrition for fall sports." http://www.eatright.org/ kids/article.aspx?id=6442460013.

19. Petrie HJ, Stover EA, and Horswill CA. "Nutritional concerns for the child and adolescent competitor." *Nutrition*. 20 (2004): 620–631.

20. Ibid.

21. Ridley K, Ainsworth BE, and Olds TS. "Development of a compendium of energy expenditures for youth." *Int J Behav Nutr Phys Act*. 10 (2008): 45.

22. Piaget, J. and Inhelder, B. *The Psychology of the Child*. 2000. New York: Basic Books.

23. Dobbs D. "Beautiful Teenage Brains." *National Geographic*. October, 2011.

24. Erikson, E. *Childhood and Society*. New York: W.W. Norton & Company, 1950.

25. Bowker A. "The relationship between sports participation and self-esteem during early adolescence." *Can J Behav Sci*. 38 (2006): 214–229.

26. Babiss LA, and Gangwisch JE. "Sports participation as a protective factor against depression and suicidal ideation in adolescents as mediated by self-esteem and social support." *J Dev Behav Peds*. 30 (2009): 376–384.

CHAPTER 2

The Starting Lineup: Major Nutrients

You are what you eat.
—Victor Lindlahr, nutritionist and author

When 16-year-old Madison gained weight during her summer break, she vowed to lose it fast when she started the season again in the fall. Her off-season weight gain was par for the course—she wasn't working out and hadn't taken a break in the eating department. Her quick-fix solution, as for many people trying to lose weight, was to cut carbs. Rather than eat less, make smarter food choices, and let exercise do the weight-loss deed, Madison went after the crucial nutrient needed by every athlete—carbohydrates—and eventually cutting out that key nutrient blunted her track performance.

Young athletes need a team of nutrients, including carbohydrates, protein, and fat—a trio that nutritionists call macronutrients—to perform best. Eliminating one will lead to suboptimal athletic performance, either immediately or down the road.

I like to think of the macronutrients as the components of a house. Carbs, which should make up at least half the calories in an athlete's diet, are the foundation of the house, providing stability, strength, and a sturdy foundation. Protein, a key to building new tissue and repairing damaged muscles, are the bricks and mortar, forming the structure and holding it all together. And fat, which cushions organs and "moisturizes" the brain, is the plumbing and electricity, providing functionality and warmth. Without any one of these components you don't have a full-fledged home.

The same is true regarding carbohydrates, protein, and fat in the young athlete's diet: if you don't include all three in balance, you won't have a well-nourished, optimally fueled body.

In this chapter, you will learn about the function of each macronutrient, how much your athlete needs, what happens when he or she doesn't get enough, and the foods that supply the best sources of each. You will also learn the reasons for nutrient recommendations for young athletes.

Busting the Myths about Carbohydrates

One of the biggest myths about nutrition and sports is that you can be cavalier with carbohydrates—that you can ignore them, give them short shrift, or, even worse, avoid them. The joke is on you if you buy into this myth because carbs are the single most important nutrient for an athlete and the cornerstone of a sports nutrition plan.

Part of the reason for the negative press for carbohydrates comes from their abuse by young and old, athlete and nonathlete. We're told to eat a diet rich in good carbs—foods like fruit, vegetables, whole grains, and dairy—but the reality is that we eat too many desserts, snacks, and sugary beverages. And kids and teens are some of the worst culprits. Too many of these foods can promote excess weight gain, which may contribute to the development of long-term diseases. Because of this, carbs are feared and have been lumped into the category of "bad for you."

Carbohydrate Control

Did you know that your brain relies on carbohydrates to function properly? The brain needs a minimum level of carbs to work well: at least 130 grams per day.

All carbohydrate food sources are digested and broken down into smaller energy bits called glucose. Glucose is present in the bloodstream (where it is known as blood sugar) and circulates to the organs, muscles, and brain, where it provides energy to the cells for proper functioning. Glucose that reaches the brain helps in such functions as concentrating and making decisions. When sufficient carbohydrates are not available, thinking gets foggy, and we may make poor decisions or have a tough time focusing. The brain cannot store glucose, so it needs a consistent and reliable source.

Our bodies can connect glucose bits into longer chains (called glycogen) for storage in the liver and muscles. We can think of these long chains of glycogen as a pearl necklace; the units of glucose are like the individual pearls. During exercise, glycogen is called upon when the body needs energy and there isn't enough in the bloodstream or from food. The glycogen chains are broken, one "pearl" at a time, to provide glucose to the bloodstream.

All the cells in the body need glucose in order to work. Because the body needs a constant supply, it keeps a tight control on the glucose from foods that are eaten and taps into those stored sources of glycogen from the muscles and the liver, as needed.

Children are limited in their ability to store carbohydrates in muscle and don't build up large stores of glycogen like adults do.[1] Females, specifically, store fewer carbs than males.[2] Accordingly, young athletes are cautioned against "loading" with carbohydrates before exercising or competition.[3] Rather, you want to encourage your athlete to eat a high-carbohydrate diet consisting of 45% to 65% of calories every day.

"Kids know that carbs are important for sports performance," says Christine Rosenbloom, PhD, RD, and a professor emeritus at Georgia State University, "but they don't know how many are contained in their favorite foods, so it is easy for them to overconsume them." For example, one slice of bread (1 oz [28 g]) is a serving. A 12-inch restaurant roll is 164 grams or *almost six servings* of bread, yet many young athletes will say about their Subway lunch, "I had one serving of bread."

Table 2-1 details the portion sizes and carbohydrate content of selected foods.

Sweets are often to blame for an excess of carbs in a young athlete's diet. From concession choices at sporting events to sweets available at home, it's easy for consumption of treats to get out of control. Ideally, these foods should be kept to a healthy average of one or two normal

Table 2-1 Carbohydrate Content of Food

Food	15 grams	20 grams	25 grams	50 grams
Dairy				
Yogurt (plain)	1⅓ cup (308 mL)	1¾ cup (414 mL)	~ 2⅓ cup (544 mL)	4⅓ cup (1017 mL)
Yogurt (flavored)	⅓ cup (71 mL)	~ ½ cup (119 mL)	–	~ 1 cup (237 mL)
Low-fat milk	~ 1 cup (237 mL)	–	~ 2 cup (474 mL)	~ 4 cup (948 mL)
Chocolate milk	~ ⅔ cup (159 mL)	¾ cup (177 mL)	~ 1 cup (237 mL)	~ 2 cup (474 mL)
Pudding	¼ cup (59 mL)	⅓ cup (71 mL)	–	~ 1 cup (237 mL)
Fruit				
Apple	½ large (3.23-inch) (111 g)	1 small (2.75-inch) (149 g)	1 medium (3-inch) (182 g)	2 medium (364 g)
Banana	½ large (8-inch) (68 g)	–	¾ large (102 g)	~ 1¾ large (238 g)
Cuties (clementines)	~2 (148 g)	–	~ 3 (222 g)	~ 5 (370 g)
Grapes	17 grapes (41 g)	22 grapes (53 g)	29 grapes (70 g)	56 grapes (134 g)
Fruit cup (packed in juice)	¾ cup (114 g)	1 cup (151 g)	1¼ cup (189 g)	2½ cup (379 g)
Vegetables				
Baby carrots	12 (180 g)	16 (240 g)	20 (300 g)	40 (600 g)
Bell peppers	1½ pepper (246 g)	2 peppers (328 g)	2½ peppers (410 g)	5 peppers (820 g)
Cucumbers	1½ cucumber (452 g)	2 (602 g)	2⅓ (692 g)	4½ (1355 g)
Edamame (in pod)	1 cup (201 g)	1½ cup (302 g)	2 cup (402 g)	6½ cup (1307 g)
Grains				
Pretzel twists	3 twists (18 g)	4 twists (24 g)	5 twists (30 g)	10 twists (60 g)
Granola bar, chewy	¾ bar (18 g)	1 bar (24 g)	1⅓ bar (31 g)	2½ bars (60 g)
Bagel (3½–4" diameter)	¼ bagel (26 g)	⅓ bagel (35 g)	½ bagel (52 g)	~ 1 bagel (105 g)
Baked chips	18 chips (22 g)	24 chips (29 g)	29 chips (35 g)	59 chips (70 g)
Cereal (i.e., honey nut cheerios)	½ cup (19 g)	¾ cup (28 g)	~1 cup (37 g)	1¾ cup (65 g)

Source: USDA Nutrient Database.[4]

portion sizes each day. One of the health hazards of eating too many sweet treats is that they often combine too many carbs with too much fat.

Yes, those ice cream cones, cookies, brownies, and coffee drinks pack some serious sugar and fat, which may mean too many calories, full tummies, and lackluster athletic performance. Sugar can be cleaned up with a trade-off system: a sweet treat on exercise days is fine, but be careful with biggies, ventis, or double dips. A single serving size should equal one sweet treat. No exercise? Try to skip the sweet treat.

When young athletes eat too many sweets, the excess carbs can be manufactured into fat and stored in fat cells, particularly if the body doesn't burn them off during exercise. Over time, the fat accumulates and may cause unwanted weight gain. Most athletes who exercise regularly and eat a wide variety of foods don't have this problem, but difficulties can arise when training stops.

The obvious antidote to overdosing on carbs is to understand which carbohydrate sources are the best and how much of them your athlete should eat. "Knowledge of portion sizes and knowing what their [carbohydrate] needs are at different times of the season is the answer," confirms Rosenbloom. I'll discuss carbohydrate needs below and help you with portions in Chapter 5.

Yes, overindulging in sweets and carbs can cause weight gain and dulled performance. Yet we know from recent research that both female and male athletes often fall short on carb consumption, especially *during* exercise, with only 18% of boys and 29% of girls matching the targets outlined below.[5] As I emphasized at the beginning, carbs supply the body with important sources of glucose and glycogen so that it can do its daily work—exercising, thinking, and learning.

While your athlete has more leeway for carbohydrates when playing sports, the key is to balance eating with exercise. When the balance is off, there may be negative effects—under-fueled muscles and low energy when carbohydrate intake is sparse, or weight gain that's hard for athletes to move around when too many carbs are consumed.

Carve Out Your Carbohydrates

There are two main types of carbohydrates: simple and complex. Simple carbohydrates consist of glucose—that basic "pearl" of energy. Because they are in their simplest form, simple carbohydrates enter the blood-stream quickly, and the body doesn't have to do much to digest them. Simple carbohydrate foods include sugar, syrup, honey, agave, high-fructose corn syrup, candy, 100% fruit juices, sports drinks, and foods made with sugar, such as most desserts.

Complex carbohydrates consist of starches and fiber-rich food sources, such as whole grains, whole fruit, vegetables, and dairy products, that require digestion to break them down to their simplest form so that they can travel to the body's cells and do their job. Digesting these complex sources is more time-consuming. During the process, small amounts of glucose are released gradually into the bloodstream—a "slow drip" that results in a steady release of energy.

Complex carbohydrate foods include fruits (such as bananas, oranges, berries, mangos, raisins, and peaches); vegetables (such as potatoes, corn, broccoli, green beans, and carrots); grains (such as breads, crackers, pasta, rice, and cereal); and dairy products (such as milk, yogurt, cheese, and cottage cheese).

Table 2-2 gives you an idea of the range of foods containing carbohydrates.

Young athletes can use both sources of carbohydrate for their benefit. Simple carbs like the ones found in 100% fruit juices or sports drinks can "top off the tank," helping your athlete get ready for competitions and stay fueled during them. On the other hand, complex carbohydrate foods, because they are digested more slowly, provide your athlete with staying power during extended exercise. They should be a key part of the training diet—foods that are eaten on a regular basis. They play a role in preparing the athlete for exercise, competition, and recovery.

The Importance of Fiber

As a serious lacrosse player, 16-year-old Danny thought he had a fairly good balance in his diet when it came to carbohydrates—no sodas and few sweets. But Danny wasn't eating enough fruits, veggies, and whole grains, and as a result he had an embarrassing issue with constipation. Kudos to Danny for nixing the sweets and soda, but he still had a lot of tweaks he needed to make to his diet. He needed a clear idea of which foods contain carbohydrates, an understanding of how they shake out with

Table 2-2 Common Foods and Their Carbohydrate Content*

Food Group	Type	Serving Size	Carb Count (grams)
Grains	Bread	1 slice (28 g)	15
	Bun	Hotdog, whole (42 g)	20
		Hamburger, whole (42 g)	20
	Pita	1 round, 2 ounces (56 g)	30
	Crackers, saltine	1 cracker (3 g)	2
	Pasta, cooked	1 cup (~150 g)	40
	Rice, other grains (barley, quinoa)	1 cup (~150 g)	45
	Dry cereal	1 cup (varies)	15–45 (check label)
	Cooked cereal	1 cup (234 g)	30
Dairy	Milk or milk alternative (soy, rice)	1 cup (237 mL)	12
	Chocolate milk	1 cup (237 mL)	26
	Yogurt	1 cup (237 mL)	12–40
	Ice cream	½ cup (119 mL)	20
Fruit	Fresh, whole	4 ounce (112 g)	15
		6 ounce (168 g)	25
		8 ounce (224 g)	35
	Canned	½ cup (119 g)	15
	Dried	1 ounce (28 g)	15
	100% juice	½ cup (119 mL)	12–20
Vegetable	Starchy		
	-Corn	½ cup (75 g)	15
	-Potato	Small (3 ounces) (84 g)	15
	-Beans	1 cup (172 g)	30–45
	Nonstarchy (greens, broccoli)	½ cup (75 g)	5
	100% juice	½ cup (119 mL)	6
Desserts, confections, and beverages	Apple pie	1 slice (1 ounce) (28 g)	10
	Cookie, Oreo	3 (25 g)	26
	Cake, chocolate, no frosting	1 slice (1/12 of cake) (95 g)	51
	Candy	Skittles, 2 ounce bag (62 g)	52
	Soda	12 ounces (356 mL)	35

*Carbohydrate content varies based on brand names and portion size; always read the label for portion size and carbohydrate content.
Sources: USDA ChooseMyPlate.gov. and USDA National Nutrient Database for Standard Reference (http://ndb.nal.usda.gov/)

regard to simple versus complex sources, and a plan for boosting fiber in his diet.

According to the 2015 Dietary Guidelines for Americans (DGA), fiber is a nutrient of public health concern for most children and teens; consumption rates for these groups are well below suggested levels.[6] The fiber found in foods such as beans, peas, fruit, vegetables, whole grains, and nuts are associated with curtailing the risk of obesity, cardiovascular disease, and type 2 diabetes. Fiber is a nondigestible form of carbohydrate; as such, it adds bulk and promotes regularity in bowel movements.

The usual intake of fiber for the average American is only 15 grams per day.[7] Young athletes need about 14 grams of fiber for every 1,000 calories they consume. Based on the calorie requirements outlined in Chapter 1, a 9-year-old gymnast who weighs 65 pounds (29.5 kg) will need about 1,800 calories per day and 25 grams of fiber. Older athletes need more calories and more fiber. You can help your young athletes meet their fiber requirements by providing high-fiber sources for them to eat throughout the day. In general, fresh fruit and veggies, whole grains and beans, and nuts and seeds contain the most fiber.

Here are some excellent sources of fiber, noted in grams (g) per serving: ½ cup (91 g) of beans such as navy, black, pinto (6–10 g); ⅓ cup (21 g) of 100% bran cereal (9 g); one medium-sized pear (5.5 g); ½ cup (73 g) of green peas (3.5–4.4 g); ½ cup (62 g) of raspberries (4.0 g); one small apple with skin (4 g); 1 ounce (28 g) of almonds (3.5 g); and one medium-sized banana (3 g).

Balancing Carbohydrates

The top priority for your young athlete should be to get the right amount of carbohydrates in his or her diet, and from the right foods—primarily complex carbohydrate sources. This means that much of the food in your athlete's diet should come from fruits, vegetables, grains, and dairy products. Only minimal amounts of high-sugar foods (desserts, soda, candy) should be eaten daily.

Once carbohydrates in the diet are in an ideal balance, the fine-tuning issues for the serious athlete become how many carbs to eat and when to eat them. Remember, pre-exercise carbohydrates help boost the glucose in the bloodstream and ready the body for optimal performance. Eating carbs during long bouts of exercise or competition helps keep the blood sugar at normal levels and offers ongoing energy "pearls" to the working muscles and brain. Post-exercise carbs help muscles recover and reload them with glycogen for the next exercise session.

Here are specific carbohydrate recommendations for the serious or elite young athlete, including guidance for daily intake and during seasonal exercise. If your athlete is a recreational one, stick with the aforementioned guidelines of 45% to 65% of daily calories from carbohydrate-based foods.

- *Low-intensity exercise or skill-based activity*[8]: 1.3 to 2.3 grams per pound per day (3–5 g/kg)
- *Moderate exercise* (1 hour per day)[9]: 2.3 to 3.2 grams of carbohydrate per pound (5–7 g/kg)
- *Endurance training* (1 to 3 hours per day)[10]: 2.7 to 4.5 grams per pound per day (6–10 g/kg)
- *Extreme training program* (4 to 5 hours per day)[11]: 3.6 to 5.5 grams per pound per day (8–12 g/kg)

Children generally fall into the low-intensity, moderate, or endurance-training categories, while elite adolescent athletes may need a higher carbohydrate diet related to their more extreme training.

Competition is a different story. For some athletes, game day involves less time exercising than practice does, and for others, competition is the pinnacle of endurance exercise. Whether your little ice skater is skating for the top position in the arena or your cross-country star is participating in his or her first 10K race, understanding the guidelines for keeping your athletes' carbohydrate stores loaded and ready will help you plan their food and drink regimen. Here are some general recommendations for carbohydrate intake before, during, and after competitive events:

- *Pre-exercise or before an athletic event (1–4 hours before activity)*[12]: ½ to 2 grams of carbohydrate per pound (1–4½ g/kg)
- *During moderate to heavy exercise*:
  - *Events lasting less than 75 minutes*[13]: no added carbohydrate needed
  - *Events lasting 75 minutes to 2½ hours*[14]: 30 to 60 grams of carbohydrate per hour

- *After exercise/recovery*[15]: about ½ gram of carbohydrate per pound per hour (1 to 1.2 g/kg) for 0 to 4 hours after exercise

---

What's the Carb Prescription?

Knowing the numbers is one thing; making them come alive for your young athlete is another. The guidelines above and the examples below will help you map out your athlete's carbohydrate prescription during competitive seasons.

Ten-year-old Kate is a soccer player. She weighs an average 75 pounds (34 kg) and practices for an hour three nights per week. This classifies her as moderately active:

Kate's daily needs during season: 175 to 240 grams of carbohydrate per day

Pre-exercise or event: 40 to 150 grams

During exercise/event: none

Recovery: 40 grams per hour

Twelve-year-old Danny is an ice hockey player. He weighs an average 90 pounds (41 kg) and practices four mornings a week for an hour and a half before school. This classifies him as moderately active:

Danny's daily needs during season: 205 to 290 grams of carbohydrate per day

Pre-exercise or event: 45 to 180 grams

During exercise/event: 30 grams per hour

Recovery: 45 grams per hour

Fourteen-year-old Claire is a rower. She weighs 110 pounds (50 kg). She rows three days each week for 2 to 3 hours. This classifies her as moderately active:

Claire's daily needs during season: 250 to 350 grams of carbohydrate per day

Pre-exercise or event: 55 to 220 grams

During exercise/event: 30 to 60 grams per hour

Recovery: 55 grams per hour

Sixteen-year-old Oliver is a basketball player. He weighs an average 135 pounds (61 kg) and practices every night for 2 hours and on Saturday mornings for 3 hours. This classifies him as an endurance trainer:

Oliver's daily needs during season: 365 to 600 grams of carbohydrate per day

Pre-exercise or event: 65 to 270 grams

During exercise/event: 30 grams per hour

Recovery: 65 grams per hour

The ranges provided are flexible and should reflect the individual athlete's age, training, level and extent of competition, and appetite. See Table 2-2, above, for food ideas to cover your athlete's carb requirement.

Carbohydrates are the foundation of a young athlete's diet, from stabilizing blood sugar and providing a reliable energy supply for the muscles, to helping the athlete recover from exercise. Simple sugars offer a quick, short-acting source of energy, while complex carbohydrates offer a preferred and enduring energy source for the exercising muscles.

While carbs are an absolutely essential component of the young athlete's diet, they can't do the job of enhancing performance alone. They need a powerful helper—protein—if your young athlete is to get the most from his or her efforts.

Protein: Getting Past the Hype

Protein is a hot topic in performance nutrition. It's sometimes thought of as the miracle nutrient, reported to build muscle with every bite. There's a lot of mystery and hype around protein, but is protein magical? Or does that myth also need to be busted?

Before we can talk about the power of protein or start a collective myth-busting session, you need to understand the role protein plays in the growth and development of children and teens, as well as its part in exercise and sports. Per pound of body weight, children and teens require more protein than adults for normal growth and development. Growing athletes need a bit more to cover the muscular demands of exercise, but not as much as you may think.

Protein and Normal Growth

In the childhood nutrition world, protein is widely recognized as the building block of growth. It's made up of 20 amino acids, which can be rearranged and configured to accommodate growth needs within the body. Nine of these amino acids are considered essential: they cannot be made by the body and must be obtained from food. They include leucine, isoleucine, and valine, otherwise known as the *branched chain amino acids*. Branched-chain amino acids have been studied in the adult sports nutrition world and pronounced important for athletes; however, few of them have been studied in the younger population. I'll talk more about this in Chapter 7.

Protein in the diet of an athlete is like the bricks and mortar of a house, responsible for building new tissue (read: muscle), which gives shape and strength to the body. At the same time, it helps to repair muscle tissue damaged by exercise. Protein has a critical role in growth and development. Because children and teens are in constant growth mode during childhood, sufficient protein intake is something you always want to ensure. When children do not get enough protein in their diets over long periods of time, they experience poor growth, malnutrition, or even stunting (lack of height gain).

The Recommended Dietary Allowance (RDA) for protein for the 8- to 12-year-old child is about *½ gram of protein per pound*.[16] This daily amount depends on body weight, so the thinner child will need less protein than the huskier preteen. For the 13- to 18-year-old, the RDA for protein is a little lower: *0.4 gram per pound*.[17] Most children and teens can meet their protein requirements with two 3-ounce (89-mL) servings of lean protein each day. Two eggs in the morning, 2 ounces (59 g) of deli turkey at lunch, and 4 ounces (118 g) of lean hamburger at dinner more than cover the minimum protein needed by the growing child or teen.

Young athletes need slightly more protein than their nonathletic counterparts. This is because they're building more muscle during exercise and need to make sure they consume enough to rebuild and repair what was damaged in the process. In general, a diet that represents about 12% to 15% of calories from protein will cover the protein requirements of the young athlete. For example, an average 14-year-old boy would match his protein needs with 65 to 80 grams of protein per day, assuming his calorie requirements are 2,200 calories per day.

During the start of a sport's season, protein needs are a bit higher due to the intensified muscle building that typically takes place. To match the requirements of this phase, protein needs are about *0.7 to 0.8 gram per pound per day* (1.5–1.7 g/kg). As training moves into a maintenance phase and your athlete's body adjusts to the exercise load, protein needs drop back down to *0.5 to 0.6 gram per pound per day* (1.0–1.4 g/kg).[18]

A 2007 report using nitrogen-balance studies in healthy adolescent male soccer players confirmed this recommendation, suggesting *0.6 gram of protein per pound of body weight per day* (1.4 g/kg) to support growth and maintain protein balance.[19] Remember, the total protein needs of teen athletes will be higher than that of a child because they are in a rapid growth phase, lean muscle tissue is accumulating at a high rate, and body weight is higher at this time. For young athletes who are involved in body building, weight lifting, or another form of muscle resistance training, protein needs may be as high as *0.5 to 1.5 grams per pound per day* (1.2–3.4 g/kg).[20]

More, Less, or Just Right?

Stop worrying! Most kids and teens meet their protein requirements through their daily diet, with athletes consuming two to three times the RDA for protein.[21] Even when athletes play sports in which there's a tendency for calorie restriction, they still meet their protein requirements, eating on average about 0.7 to 0.9 gram per pound per day (1.5–2.0 g/kg).[22] Of course, some athletes may not meet their protein needs, especially those eating a plant-based diet and those who put themselves on a diet to lose weight. These athletes may require extra guidance and monitoring to make sure they get enough protein.

Table 2-3 lists typical protein sources and their protein contribution.

Mike wanted his 11-year-old soccer-playing son, Charlie, to bulk up, and brought him to me to plan out a high-protein diet to get the job done. "All Charlie eats are carbs, and I told him if he eats more protein, he'll have more muscle," Mike said. I checked Charlie's usual eating routine, and while he wasn't a big fan of meat (he didn't like the texture), he was getting plenty of protein through dairy products, eggs, lunchmeat, and nuts. I explained to both Mike and Charlie that eating more protein as a way to pack on muscle is a myth that doesn't hold water. Mike was onto something, though: protein *was* one key to muscle building. But he didn't understand that eating protein wasn't enough.

Athletes need to eat enough calories to make protein available to muscles (a concept called *protein-sparing*, which means protein is preserved and not used up as a calorie source). In addition, exercise is necessary in order to build more muscle tissue. When protein is consumed along with enough calories *and* exercise occurs, more muscle building happens, as long as the changes involved in puberty are in motion.[23] This is particularly true when exercise is resistance-based, such as in weight lifting or weight training.

Unfortunately, there's a dark side to protein that many don't understand. As with eating too many carbs, high-protein diets that go beyond an individual's need for protein and calories can cause unwanted weight gain, particularly if the person doesn't routinely engage in exercise.[24] Too much protein can also put extra stress on the kidneys and liver, promote dehydration, and result in loss of calcium (an important nutrient for bone building) in the urine. Younger children are more susceptible to kidney and liver stress than older teens because of their smaller size and physical immaturity. And don't forget that eating a lot of protein can crowd out carbohydrates, which may negatively affect athletic performance. Like all things nutrition, finding the right balance of protein for your growing athlete is the key.

In the case of Charlie, Mike needed to understand the potential outcomes of pushing too much protein. If Charlie were to eat too much, he could get too many calories and might see changes in his body fat (read:

Table 2-3 Protein Content of Selected Foods[4]

Food	Serving Size	Protein (grams)
Chicken	4 ounces (112 g)	32
Turkey	4 ounce (112 g)	34
Egg	1 large	6
Yogurt (Greek)	6 ounce (178 mL)	17
Yogurt	6 ounce (178 mL)	10
Milk	1 cup (237 mL)	8
Whey protein powder	1 scoop (45 grams)	26
Cheese	1 ounce (28 g)	7
Tuna	4 ounce (112 g)	27
Nuts	1 ounce (28 g)	5
Beans, cooked	1 cup (172 g)	6
Hummus	2 tablespoons (30 g)	2
Edamame	½ cup (78 g)	8
Soy milk	1 cup (237 mL)	7
Soy yogurt	6 ounce (178 mL)	6
Soy protein powder	1 scoop (45 grams)	26
Quinoa	1 cup (150 g)	8
Lentils	1 cup (172 g)	18
Tofu	½ cup (126 g)	20
Tempeh	½ cup (83 g)	15
Peanut butter	2 tablespoons (22 g)	8

fat gain), while increasing the risk of dehydration and stress on his kidneys. If he were to eat ample protein but miss out on sufficient calories, he might lose muscle mass. The ideal situation for Charlie was to eat a balanced diet of all foods, including protein sources like egg, deli meat, and dairy foods; make sure to eat protein at each meal; have an after-exercise protein-inclusive snack; and engage in regular bouts of resistance exercise. And, of course, wait for puberty to kick in.

Recovery: A Special Role for Protein

Protein has a special role in post-exercise recovery. Several studies of adults have shown that small doses of protein after an intense exercise session can repair muscle damage and promote muscle gain.[25] Chocolate milk has been identified as a simple way to achieve muscle repair. Its protein content of about 10 grams per cup and its carbohydrate content of 27 grams per cup help repair the muscle tissue and reload it with glycogen.

The protein source in chocolate milk is a combination of casein (the main protein found in milk, which coagulates into a curd when cheese is made) and whey (the watery part of milk that separates from the curd). Whey is considered a "fast protein" because it's quickly absorbed and available to muscles. It's also a concentrated source of leucine, an amino acid that has been shown to help adults eliminate muscle soreness after exercise and potentially enhance mental function; more studies are needed, particularly of young people.[26] I'll talk more about this supplement in Chapter 7.

The truth is, any food item that offers a combination of carbohydrate and protein may offer positive benefits to the young athlete after exercise. Eating a protein-carbohydrate food combination *within 45 minutes* of exercise completion will improve the body's ability to repair and restore muscles.[27]

---

15 Protein-containing Snacks to Eat After Exercise

1. 8 to 10 ounces (237 to 296 mL) of chocolate milk
2. 8 ounces (237 mL) of bottled or homemade yogurt smoothie drink
3. Mozzarella cheese stick and four wheat crackers
4. Single-serve peanut butter cup (2 tablespoons [30 g]) and one to two sheets (four to eight rectangles) of graham crackers
5. Small banana and 6 ounces (177 mL) of Greek yogurt
6. 1 to 2 ounces (28 to 57 g) of beef or turkey jerky and four whole-grain crackers
7. ⅔ cup (104 g) of edamame with fresh veggies
8. ½ cup (70 g) nuts and dried fruit mix

9. ½ to ¾ cup (70 to 105 g) trail mix with nuts/seeds
10. 1 cup (140 g) yogurt and 2 tablespoons (30 g) dried fruit
11. Half a cheese sandwich (one or two slices of cheese)
12. Half a peanut-butter-and-jelly sandwich
13. Single-serve tuna pack with four to six crackers
14. Liquid meal supplement
15. Granola bar (containing 10 g of protein)

Striking the Balance

Balancing protein in the diet is an important task for young athletes, particularly in light of common teen eating patterns, which may not feature much protein. If your athletes get most of their nutrition at the end of the day or after school, something I call "back-loading," they may be under-eating protein (and carbohydrates) throughout the day and getting too many calories. The goal is to have a consistent supply of nutrients available to the muscles so that they are primed and ready for exercise, a balance that is best achieved by serving meals and providing snacks at regular times.

Leslie Bonci is a sports dietitian for the National Football League, the National Hockey League, Major League Baseball, the Women's National Basketball Association, and the Ladies Professional Golf Association, and director of sports nutrition at the University of Pittsburgh Medical Center. She says that young athletes make three mistakes with protein:

- They rely on supplements like powders and shakes instead of food.
- They unevenly distribute protein throughout the day (often eating none at breakfast, some at lunch, and a lot at dinner).
- They experiment with vegetarianism and remove protein from the plate.

Instead, Bonci advises young athletes to use *food* as the primary protein source and to evenly distribute it, making sure to have at least some with their breakfast, lunch, dinner, and snacks. I'll detail how you can spread out the protein in Chapter 5.

Fat Can Be Your Friend

Whether you are pro-fat, anti-fat, or somewhere in between, when it comes to young athletes, fat can be a friend indeed. It's the highest calorie-containing nutrient in the diet, hosting a whopping 9 calories per gram, more than twice the calories of carbohydrates and protein. If your athlete isn't careful, fat can wreck his or her diet, encourage weight gain, and curtail athletic performance.

This happened to Tom, who got his driver's license and started to spend a lot of time eating out. His daily drive-by snacks after football practice gained him an empty wallet and a robust waistline. Not surprisingly, teen athletes like Tom may fall prey to the freedom that comes with driving and semi-adulthood. If these freedoms are abused, they can negatively impact both weight status and athletic performance.

But fat isn't always the bad guy. It can be an asset, too, particularly if calorie needs are high or a little extra weight on the frame is needed. Adding fat, especially if your athlete doesn't like to eat huge amounts of food, can help. Rather than being afraid of fat and becoming extreme about it—eliminating it, overdoing it, or simply making the wrong choices—learn how to use this nutrient to your athlete's benefit. But, first, a little background information.

What Does Fat Do?

Fat helps the body absorb certain nutrients, particularly the fat-soluble nutrients vitamin A, vitamin D, vitamin E, and vitamin K. It also offers important essential fatty acids, such as omega-3 fatty acids, and acts as a cushion around the internal organs, protecting them from injury. Fat has an important role in brain growth and function as well, helping provide structure (the brain is almost 60% fat) and facilitating communication within the brain. While the growth of the brain is nearly complete by age 5 or 6, fat maintains a central role in its function throughout life.

Your athlete needs a brain that can think clearly, make quick decisions, and focus, especially in the heat of the moment. Essential fatty acids—especially eicosapentaenoic acid (EPA) and docosahexaenoic acid (DHA), also known as omega-3 fatty acids—are healthy fats that should be included in the diet every day. EPA is responsible for brain structure and neurotransmission, and it plays a role in the immune system. Fats rich in DHA, like fish and DHA-fortified eggs, have a positive influence on visual acuity and mental development.[28]

Understanding Fat Lingo

Fats come from plants or animals or are man-made. Animal fats—such as butter, cheese, the marbling on a steak, or the skin on chicken—are *saturated fats* and are associated with the development of heart disease. Limit these foods sources to less than 10% of the calories in your athlete's diet.

Plant fats, also called *unsaturated fats*, include oils made from olives, nuts, seeds, or plants that naturally contain fat, such as avocado. Unsaturated fats can be *polyunsaturated* or *monounsaturated*, both of which are good options. Monounsaturated fatty acids (MUFAs) are among the healthiest fats to include in your athlete's diet. Olive and canola oils, peanut butter, and avocado are examples of MUFAs. *Polyunsaturated fatty acids* (PUFAs), such as salmon, soybean and corn oil, walnuts and sunflower seeds, along with MUFAs, protect against the development of heart disease. Both MUFAs and PUFAs should make up the majority of the fat in your athlete's diet.

Manufactured fats, known as *trans-fats*, are made by hydrogenating oils (infusing hydrogen into liquid fat to make it a solid fat) and are the unhealthiest fats for your young athlete's growing body. They may contribute to the development of heart disease and cancer. You'll find *trans-fats* in shelf-stable foods like crackers, cookies, and some bakery items. The American Heart Association recommends consuming less than 1% of your daily calories in the form of trans-fat, or less than 2 grams (2,000 mg) per day.[29]

Fat and Exercise

Fat is stored in the body in adipose tissue (fat tissue) and in the muscles in the form of triacylglycerol, also known as triglyceride (TG), the scientific name for fat. The fat around the outside of a nice steak is like the adipose tissue on the body; the streaks of fat within the steak are like the

TG in an athlete's muscle. Both adipose tissue and TG are banks of energy from which your athlete can draw during exercise.

In children, fat is the energy source the body prefers to use during exercise. This ability to burn fat as a fuel source is called fat oxidation.[30] Once puberty has begun, teen athletes gradually move from efficient fat use during exercise to using carbohydrates as a fuel source, like adults. By middle to late puberty, teens generally have settled in to a more grown-up metabolic pattern and rely on carbs as the preferred energy source.

However, there are several altering factors. Teens who participate in regular endurance training may adapt to using fat as a fuel source and reduce their reliance on carbohydrates.[31] While children preferentially burn fat, teens can continue to do this, especially if they acclimate to regular training and thus build up more cells in the body that burn fat. It's recommended that endurance athletes who train for more than 2 hours a day consume a minimum of *0.9 gram of fat per pound per day* to ensure adequate triglyceride stores in the muscles.[32] The bottom line is that younger children and highly trained teen athletes rely more on fat as a fuel source, and older, untrained, or recreational athletes tend to use carbohydrate as the primary energy source.

Hormones also play a role and can affect the fuel source used by young athletes, especially young women who are menstruating. Fluctuating hormone levels influence the amount of fat the body uses for energy and may lead to a reduced reliance on carbohydrates.[33]

Despite all the evidence that younger athletes readily use fat as a fuel source, it is not recommended that young athletes eat more fat. Some studies have shown that high fat intake in children during exercise suppresses the release of growth hormone (the hormone responsible for overall growth and development in children and teens). Scientists believe that higher levels of growth hormone during exercise are needed for muscle growth and adaptation, so a diet that's high in fat may be counterproductive.[34]

How Much Fat Do Young Athletes Need?

As a nation, our effort to finesse fat intake is ongoing. We all know that too much fat intake is associated with overweight and obesity and can compromise athletic performance. And you may be surprised to know that even some of the leanest, fittest young athletes have considerable fat stores, despite their training.[35] Some have the same challenges as nonathletic kids and teens: high cholesterol, elevated lipid profiles, and excess weight.

The Highest-Fat Foods Consumed by Kids and Teens[36]

- *Grain-based foods*: cake, pie, cookies, donuts, crisps, cobblers, granola bars
- *Dairy-based foods*: butter, regular-fat cheese, ice cream, cream, dairy-based desserts, whole milk
- *Vegetables*: French fries
- *Meats*: sausage, franks, ribs, bacon, regular ground beef, marbled meats, poultry skin
- *Others*: chicken fat, pork fat, shortening, stick margarine

---

It's recommended that young athletes follow the national guidelines for fat intake established for children and teens by the American Heart Association and supported by other national organizations, such as the American Academy of Pediatrics (AAP) and the Academy of Nutrition and Dietetics (AND).

Young athletes should consume an amount of fat equivalent to 25% to 35% of total calories, with most fat sources coming from polyunsaturated and monounsaturated fats such as nuts, seeds, avocado, and fish. Of the fat consumed, 10% or less should come from saturated fat sources, such as butter, cheese, whole milk, and other animal fats. As noted, the consumption of trans-fats should be minimal, and cholesterol in the diet should be less than 300 milligrams per day.[37]

The easiest way to go about this is to crowd out or limit animal fats and trans-fats and to work in more plant-based fats. Simply opt for nuts, seeds, avocado, olives, olive oil, other plant oils (vegetable, canola, sunflower), peanut butter and other nut butters, ground flax seed and flax seed oil, and fatty fish (salmon, tuna, mackerel), which are full of beneficial omega-3 fatty acids.

If your young athlete is eating too much fat or is carrying too much weight, it's time to cut back on fat. In the case of overweight or obesity, experts agree that a reduction in fat intake is the way to go for children and teen athletes.[38] Decreasing fat preserves the carbohydrate and protein sources in the diet, which are needed for growth and performance. Cutting back on how much butter, fried foods, chips, and fatty desserts like ice cream your athlete eats can help prevent further weight gain and contribute to a healthy weight reduction.

Some athletes may cut out fat too aggressively. A very-low-fat diet is not healthy for growing athletes and can be a slippery slope that leads to insufficient intake of essential fatty acids and fat-soluble vitamins, and cuts out important protein-rich foods like lean meats and dairy foods. Absence of these foods in the diet may mean inadequate intake of important nutrients such as iron, zinc, and calcium.[39] In severe cases, fat elimination can be the precursor for disordered eating and even a full-blown eating disorder. I'll cover more on this topic in Chapter 9.

Rather than focus on counting fat grams, use these guidelines to help your athlete trim the fat without nixing important nutrients:

- Use olive, canola, or vegetable oil when cooking or baking.
- Serve fruits and veggies with every meal. They are fat-free and will tip the balance to lower-fat meals overall.
- Switch over to eating whole-grain foods such as 100% whole wheat bread, oats, or quinoa most of the time.
- Avoid fried foods, except for infrequent special occasions.
- Eat at home.
- Limit desserts to one reasonable serving per day or, better, a couple per week.

On the flip side, if your child or teen needs to gain weight, adding healthy fat sources like olive oil, avocado, and nuts will help provide extra calories without the need to eat mounds of food. For example, you can double-dress pasta by tossing it in olive oil first and then sauce, or add a swipe of avocado on deli-meat sandwiches to boost calories.

Young athletes need all three macronutrients—carbohydrates, protein, and fat—in their diet for top performance. De-emphasizing one or another is a dangerous practice that will eventually have consequences. The secret to getting all three, and in the right combination, is knowing the proportion of each nutrient your athlete needs, the best food sources and where to get them, and how much your athlete should eat to gain the proper fuel for training and competition. When you know these things, you'll be able to tailor training and competition diets to your athlete's needs so that he or she has a performance advantage.

Notes

1. Hoch AZ, Goossen K, and Kretschmer T. Nutritional requirements of the child and teenage athlete. *Phys Med Rehabil Clin N Am*. 19 (2008): 373–398.
2. Position of the American Dietetic Association, Dietitians of Canada, and the American College of Sports Medicine: Nutrition and Athletic Performance. *J Acad Nutr Diet*. 109 (2009): 509–527.
3. Jeukendrup A and Cronin L. "Nutrition and elite young athletes." *Med Sport Sci*. 56 (2011): 47–58.
4. U.S. Department of Agriculture, Agricultural Research Service. 2014. USDA National Nutrient Database for Standard Reference, Release 27. Nutrient Data Laboratory home page. http://www.ars.usda.gov/ba/bhnrc/ndl.
5. Baker LB, Heaton LE, Nuccio RP, and Stein KW. Dietitian-observed nutrient intakes of young skill and team-sport athletes: adequacy of pre, during, and post-exercise nutrition. *Int J Sport Nutr Exer Metab*. 24 (2014): 166–176.
6. U.S. Department of Agriculture and U.S. Department of Health and Human Services. "*Dietary Guidelines for Americans, 2015*." Available at: http://www.health.gov/dietaryguidelines/2015-scientific-report/PDFs/Scientific -Report-of-the-2015-Dietary-Guidelines-Advisory-Committee.pdf.
7. Ibid.
8. Rosenbloom C, ed. *Sports Nutrition: A Practice Manual for Professionals*, 5th ed. Chicago: Academy of Nutrition and Dietetics, 2012.
9. Desbrow B, McCormack J, Burke LM, Cox GR, Fallon K, Hislop M, Logan R, Marino N, Sawyer SM, Shaw G, Star A, Vidgen H, and Leveritt M. Sports dietitians Australia position statement: sports nutrition for the adolescent athlete. *Int J Sport Exerc Metab*. 24 (2014): 570–584.
10. Hoch et al, op. cit.
11. Rosenbloom, op. cit.
12. Hoch et al, op. cit.
13. Burke LM, Hawley JA, Wong SH, and Jeukendrup AE. "Carbohydrates for training and competition." *J Sports Sci*. 29 (2011): S17–S27.
14. Ibid.

15. Ibid.
16. Food and Nutrition Board, Institute of Medicine, National Academies. "Dietary Reference Intakes for energy, carbohydrate, fiver, fat, fatty acids, cholesterol, protein, and amino acids (macronutrients)." (2002, 2005). www.nap.edu.
17. Ibid.
18. Hoch et al, op. cit.
19. Boisseau N, Vermorel M, Rance M, Duche P, Patureau-Mirand P. "Protein requirements in male adolescent soccer players." *Eur J Appl Physiol.* 100 (2007): 27–33.
20. Hoch et al, op. cit.
21. Jeukendrup and Cronin, op. cit.
22. Ibid.
23. Phillips SM, Tang JE, and Moore DM. "The role of milk- and soy-based protein in support of muscle protein synthesis and muscle protein accretion in young and elderly persons." *J Am Coll Nutr.* 28 (2009): 343–354.
24. Nemet D and Eliakim A. "Pediatric sports nutrition: an update." *Curr Opin Clin Nutr Metab Care.* 12 (2009): 304–309.
25. Jeukendrup and Cronin, op. cit.
26. Campbell B, Kreider RB, Ziegenfuss T, La Bounty P, Roberts M, Burke D, Landis J, Lopez H, and Antonio J. International Society of Sports Nutrition position stand: protein and exercise. *J Int Soc Sports Nutr.* 4 (2007): 8.
27. Kerksick C, Harvey T, Stout J, Campbell B, Wilborn C, Kreider R, Kalman D, Ziegenfuss T, Lopez H, Landis J, Ivy JL, and Antonio J. International Society of Sports Nutrition position stand: nutrient timing. *J Int Soc Sports Nutr.* 5 (2008): 17.
28. Chang CY, Ke DS, and Chen JY. Essential fatty acids and human brain. *Acta Neurol Taiwan.* 18 (2009): 231–241.
29. American Heart Association. "Fats 101." http://www.heart.org/HEART ORG/GettingHealthy/FatsAndOils/Fats101/Trans-Fats_UCM_301120 _Article.jsp.
30. Meyer F, O'Connor H, Shirreffs SM, and the International Association of Athletics Federations. "Nutrition for the young athlete." *J Sports Sci.* 25 (2007): S73–S82.
31. Shaw CS, Clark J, and Wagenmakers AJ. "The effect of exercise and nutrition on intramuscular fat metabolism and insulin sensitivity." *Annu Rev Nutr.* 30 (2010): 13–34.
32. Stellingwerff T, Maughan RJ, and Burke LM. "Nutrition for power sports: middle-distance running, track cycling, rowing, canoeing/kayaking and swimming." *J Sports Sci.* 29 (2011): S79–S89.

33. Tarnopolsky LJ, MacDougall JD, Atkinson SA, Tarnopolsky MA, and Sutton JR. "Gender differences in substrate for endurance exercise." *J Appl Physio.* 68 (1990): 302–306.
34. American Heart Association, op. cit.
35. Hoch et al, op. cit.
36. Reedy J and Krebs-Smith SM. "Dietary sources of energy, solid fats, and added sugars among children and adolescents in the United States." *J Am Diet Assoc.* 110 (2010): 1477–1484.
37. American Heart Association. Dietary recommendations for healthy children. http://www.heart.org/HEARTORG/GettingHealthy/NutritionCenter/Dietary-Recommendations-for-Healthy-Children_UCM_303886_Article.jsp.
38. Jeukendrup and Cronin, op. cit.
39. Petrie HJ, Stover EA, and Horswill CA. "Nutritional concerns for the child and adolescent competitor." *Nutrition.* 20 (2004): 620–631.

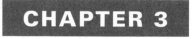

CHAPTER 3

The Second String: Vitamins and Minerals

Simplicity is the most important thing, especially when you're training.
—Garrett Weber-Gale, two-time Olympic gold medalist in swimming

Sixteen-year-old Trish was driving herself into the ground. She was constantly fatigued and couldn't seem to get enough rest. During training she was often breathless and light-headed. Her dad came to me with his concerns. "Trish just started rowing a year ago, and at the same time she decided to be a vegan," he said. "I've supported her all the way, but over the last 2 or 3 months I've watched her deteriorate. Honestly, she'd become so healthy, I can't understand what's happening." He told me that when Trish visited her doctor she learned she was iron-deficient. Trish didn't realize that in her efforts to "go vegan," she was missing out on good iron sources and derailing both her health and her endurance in a grueling sport.

Many families, athletes, and coaches forget about vitamins and minerals, also known as micronutrients. Or they don't understand that vitamins and minerals are key players in the metabolic function of the body, helping it to use the food we eat. They complement the starting lineup of carbohydrates, protein, and fat, acting as cofactors so the body can process food efficiently. When young athletes reduce their intake of one or several of them, a deficiency can occur, causing health problems that can get in the way of their growth and performance.

In this chapter, you'll learn about the function of vitamins and minerals in the human body, as well as the recommended daily requirement for the young athlete. You'll learn about the important micronutrients for the young athlete—iron, calcium, vitamin D, and others. You'll learn to recognize an "at risk" athlete, so you can be ready to intervene should you suspect a problem. As you've grown to expect from this book, I stress a well-balanced diet and will recommend decision factors for whether you should start micronutrient supplementation—one of the most commonly used (and overused) antidotes to a marginal diet.

The Purpose and Function of Vitamins and Minerals

For many people, vitamins and minerals are a mysterious part of nutrition. Most recognize their importance to a healthy diet but are unsure of their purposes and functions. It doesn't help that there are roughly 14 vitamins and over 22 minerals to stay on top of. Thankfully, you don't have to drive yourself crazy remembering each and every one. I will explain the ones that are most critical for the growth, development, and health of your athlete.

Collectively, vitamins and minerals are referred to as micronutrients, or small nutrients. They differ from carbohydrates, protein, and fat—the macronutrients—in that they do not supply calories. Rather, each micronutrient has a specific job to do in the body that relates to maintaining your athlete's health and supporting his or her growth and development.

Vitamins are made by plants or animals, and are divided into two types: fat-soluble and water-soluble vitamins. The fat-soluble vitamins, which include vitamins A, D, E, and K, are responsible for a variety of functions, such as bone health, muscle movement, blood clotting, and vision. Fat-soluble vitamins can be stored within the body, and in high dosages they may become toxic.

Water-soluble vitamins include the B vitamins (riboflavin, thiamin, niacin, pantothenic acid, folic acid, vitamin B_6, and vitamin B_{12}), biotin, choline, and vitamin C. They are not stored in the body, which means your athlete needs to get these from food sources. Generally, if someone eats more of a water-soluble vitamin than is needed, it is eliminated from the body, mostly through the urine.

Minerals come from the soil or water, are absorbed by plants or eaten by animals, and thus enter our food supply. There are a lot of minerals, some familiar and some not so familiar. The minerals calcium, chloride, chromium, copper, fluoride, iodine, iron, magnesium, manganese, molybdenum, phosphorus, potassium, selenium, sodium, sulfur, and zinc all play key roles in our bodies.

Minerals have many functions—in the health of bones and teeth, energy production and regulation, nerve and muscle function, and immunity, to name a few. Some, like calcium, are needed in large amounts on a daily basis, while others, like iron, a trace mineral, are needed in smaller amounts. Most vitamins and minerals cannot be produced by the body and must be obtained from food or from a vitamin and mineral supplement. Exceptions include vitamin D, which is generated in the skin through sun exposure; vitamin K; and some B vitamins, which can be produced in the intestinal tract.

The minimum amount of each vitamin and mineral that the body needs, called the Recommended Dietary Allowance (RDA), is based on a person's age and sex.[1] The Adequate Intake (AI) is an amount generally regarded as sufficient to meet the body's requirements for growth and health. Table 3-1 gives the RDA or the AI for selected micronutrients for children and teens.

Many micronutrients have a threshold, or saturation, level in our bodies. Once that threshold is met, the excess vitamin or mineral may become toxic. For instance, too much vitamin B_6 can cause sensory neuropathy, a condition in which the control of bodily movements is lost.[2] In the case of fat-soluble vitamins, which are stored in body tissue and organs, toxicity can be a real concern. An example is vitamin A toxicity, which can lead to vision changes, bone pain, and, in severe cases, liver damage.

For every micronutrient there is an established ceiling called the tolerable upper limit (UL). Beyond this limit, the danger of toxicity is real. As important as it is to make sure your growing athlete is getting *enough* vitamins and minerals, it is equally critical to ensure that he or she is not

(text continues on page 70)

Table 3-1 Selected Micronutrients

Micronutrient	Age (years)	RDA/AI	UL	Sources
Iron	8 9–13 14–18	10 mg 8 mg 11 mg (male) 15 mg (female)	40 mg 40 mg 45 mg 45 mg	Breakfast cereals fortified with iron; white beans; dark chocolate; hummus; lentils; spinach; tofu; beef; baked potato; cashews; chicken; whole wheat bread; raisins; egg
Calcium	8 9–13 14–18	1,000 mg 1,300 mg 1,300 mg (male) 1,300 mg (female)	2,500 mg 3,000 mg 3,000 mg 3,000 mg	Plain yogurt; mozzarella cheese; cheddar cheese; milk; soymilk; fortified orange juice; tofu; cottage cheese; canned salmon; ready-to-eat cereals; raw kale; vanilla ice cream; bok choy; broccoli
Vitamin D	8 9–13 14–18	600 IU 600 IU 600 IU (male) 600 IU (female)	3,000 IU 4,000 IU 4,000 IU 4,000 IU	Cod liver oil; swordfish; salmon; canned tuna fish; fortified orange juice; fortified milk; yogurt; egg; ready-to-eat cereals
Vitamin B$_{12}$	8 9–13 14–18	1.2 µg 1.8 µg 2.4 µg (male) 2.4 µg (female)	Not determined Not determined Not determined Not determined	Beef liver; clams; fish; beef; poultry; eggs; milk and other dairy products; some breakfast cereals; nutritional yeast
Folate	8 9–13 14–18	200 µg 300 µg 400 µg (male) 400 µg (female)	400 µg 600 µg 800 µg 800 µg	Beef liver; spinach; black-eye peas; fortified breakfast cereals; rice; asparagus; avocado; bread

(continues)

Table 3-1 (continued)

Micronutrient	Age (years)	RDA/AI	UL	Sources
Vitamin B$_6$	8 9–13 14–18	0.6 mg 1 mg 1.3 mg (male) 1.2 mg (female)	40 mg 60 mg 80 mg 80 mg	Chick peas; beef liver; tuna; salmon; chicken breast; breakfast cereals; potatoes; turkey; banana; spaghetti sauce; waffles; bulgur; cottage cheese
Thiamin	8 9–13 14–18	0.6 mg 0.9 mg 1.2 mg (male) 1.0 mg (female)	Not determined Not determined Not determined Not determined	Lentils; green peas; brown rice; white rice; enriched bread; fortified breakfast cereals; wheat germ; pork; pecans; spinach; orange; canta-loupe; milk; egg
Riboflavin	8 9–13 14–18	0.6 mg 0.9 mg 1.3 mg (male) 1.0 mg (female)	Not determined Not determined Not determined Not determined	Milk; cheddar cheese; egg; almonds; salmon; halibut; chicken; beef; broccoli; asparagus; spinach
Niacin	8 9–13 14–18	8 mg 12 mg 16 mg (male) 14 mg (female)	15 mg 20 mg 30 mg 30 mg	Yeast; chicken; tuna; turkey; salmon; beef; breakfast cereals; peanuts; pasta; lentils; lima beans; bread; coffee
Vitamin C	8 9–13 14–18	25 mg 45 mg 75 mg (male) 65 mg (female)	650 mg 1,200 mg 1,800 mg 1,800 mg	Fruits and vegetables; ready-to-eat cereals
Vitamin A	8 9–13 14–18	400 µg 600 µg 900 µg (male) 700 µg (female)	900 µg 1,700 µg 2,800 µg 2,800 µg	Milk; eggs; leafy green vegetables; orange and yellow vegetables; tomato products; some vegetable oils; fortified ready-to-eat cereals

Micronutrient	Age (years)	RDA/AI	UL	Sources
Vitamin E	8 9–13 14–18	7 mg 11 mg 15 mg (male) 15 mg (female)	300 mg 600 mg 800 mg 800 mg	Wheat germ oil; sunflower seeds; almonds; sunflower and safflower oils; peanut butter; spinach; broccoli; kiwifruit; mango; tomato
Zinc	8 9–13 14–18	5 mg 8 mg 11 mg (male) 9 mg (female)	12 mg 23 mg 34 mg 34 mg	Oysters; beef; crab; fortified breakfast cereal; lobster; pork; baked beans; chicken; yogurt; oatmeal; almonds
Selenium	8 9–13 14–18	30 µg 40 µg 55 µg (male) 55 µg (female)	150 µg 280 µg 400 µg 400 µg	Seafood; organ meats; breakfast cereals; other grains; dairy products; Brazil nuts; enriched macaroni; ham; cottage cheese; brown rice; egg; whole wheat bread; bananas
Magnesium	8 9–13 14–18	130 mg 240 mg 410 mg (male) 360 mg (female)	110 mg 350 mg 350 mg 350 mg	Green leafy vegetables; spinach; almonds; cashews; peanuts; seeds; black beans; edamame; breakfast cereals; whole wheat bread

Abbreviations: AI, Adequate Intake; RDA, Recommended Dietary Allowance; UL, upper limit.
Sources: Adapted from Dietary Reference Intakes for Calcium, Phosphorus, Magnesium, Vitamin D, and Fluoride (1997); Dietary Reference Intakes for Thiamin, Riboflavin, Niacin, Vitamin B_6, Folate, Vitamin B_{12}, Pantothenic Acid, Biotin, and Choline (1998); Dietary Reference Intakes for Vitamin C, Vitamin E, Selenium, and Carotenoids (2000); Dietary Reference Intakes for Vitamin A, Vitamin K, Arsenic, Boron, Chromium, Copper, Iodine, Iron, Manganese, Molybdenum, Nickel, Silicon, Vanadium, and Zinc (2001); Dietary Reference Intakes for Energy, Carbohydrate, Fiber, Fat, Fatty Acids, Cholesterol, Protein, and Amino Acids (2002/2005); and Dietary Reference Intakes for Calcium and Vitamin D (2011). Available at: http://fnic.nal.usda.gov/dietary-guidance/dietary -reference-intakes/dri-tables-and-application-reports

getting *too much*. Most athletes will be safe with intake amounts equivalent to the RDA, but should not take more than twice the RDA.[3] The UL for many vitamins and minerals are shown in Table 3-1.

Micronutrients offer a variety of benefits to young athletes, both for their overall growth and development, and to enhance their athletic performance. For example, calcium and vitamin D are required for bone growth and development. Deficiencies in these micronutrients during the growing years may cause stress fractures, and in adulthood they may result in osteoporosis. Most people are aware that vitamin C helps the immune system stay strong, but other micronutrients—such as vitamins A and E, zinc, and selenium—also help keep it robust.

Today's children and teens are falling behind on their consumption of dairy products, fruits, and vegetables, which supply some of the critical nutrients needed by growing athletes. In fact, few children and teens are meeting the Estimated Average Requirements (EAR) or AI of calcium, vitamin D, potassium, and fiber.[4] Teens, in particular, have higher nutrient needs due to their accelerated growth. Iron, an important nutrient for the teen athlete, especially girls, is one of the most common nutrient deficits.[5] Unhealthy eating habits like skipping breakfast can complicate the situation further.

Exercise ramps up your athlete's metabolism and may magnify nutrient inadequacies. When young athletes become deficient in micronutrients, premature fatigue and an inability to maintain a heavy training load are likely to set in.[6] Shortages of calcium can cause muscles to cramp, and iron deficits can cause shortness of breath. These difficulties may become problematic during practices and competitions and, if they persist, can lead to serious problems like poor bone density and iron deficiency anemia.

Critical Vitamins and Minerals for the Young Athlete

As you've already learned, growth and sports place a unique demand on the young athlete. Growth requires more consumption of nutrients such as calcium and iron because there is a higher need for them (calcium for bones) or because greater losses occur at this stage of life (iron in menstruating females). Some sports, such as distance running, can involve tightly controlled eating patterns, like restricting certain foods or becoming highly selective with eating times, and these can negatively impact a young athlete's nutritional status.

Eighteen-year-old Maggie, a gymnast, was very controlled in the foods she would eat and when she would eat them. She was naturally tall and slim, but when she turned 16, she started to fill out and began to eliminate more and more foods in order to maintain her thin, muscular figure. She rarely ate desserts, fast food, "white foods" such as rice or pasta, or anything else she deemed unhealthy. She wouldn't eat after 6 p.m. and kept her food intake to three meals a day, and no snacks. For the most part, Maggie survived on fish, vegetables, fruit, and water or hot tea. Her pediatrician sent her to me for a nutrition evaluation, especially in light of a recent blood test that showed a low iron level. It turned out that, yes, Maggie's diet was low in iron, and it was also lacking in other nutrients. And because her eating habits had gotten so extreme, she was flirting with developing an eating disorder.

Don't let your child or teen's healthy body weight or normal appearance fool you. Even though young athletes may look healthy, they may be missing critical nutrients in their diet. Amy Culp, a registered dietitian and the sports RD for the University of Texas, commonly sees these three micronutrient mistakes among her collegiate athletes:

- Long-term inadequate intake of calcium and iron, leading to poor bone and overall health
- A gradual reduction in dairy intake over the years, leading to an insufficient quality and quantity of calcium in the diet
- Consumption of a limited variety of foods, which negatively impacts exposure to needed micronutrients.

"Athletes should target nutrient-rich foods at every meal and snack, especially those foods containing calcium and iron," says Culp. She suggests chocolate milk or dried fruit and calcium-fortified dry cereal after intense exercise, and a nutrient-packed breakfast every day. Sports nutritionists such as Amy and I can make these recommendations all day long, but if you don't understand *why* we make them, they'll fall from your priority list. Let's investigate in more detail the critical nutrients that you should keep in mind.

Iron

Iron carries oxygen in the blood, shuttling it to the organs and to cells throughout the body, which need oxygen to function properly. The red blood cells are the star players responsible for getting oxygen from the lungs to the organs. You can imagine how important this oxygen-carrying capacity is to athletes.

Iron has two forms: *heme iron*, which comes from meat, poultry, and fish; and *nonheme iron,* which comes from plant-based foods and fortified foods. Heme iron from animals is more bioavailable (easier to absorb and utilize) than nonheme iron from plant sources. Meat, fish, poultry, and sources of vitamin C increase the absorption of nonheme iron. Additionally, phytates, compounds found in whole grains, beans, and seeds, can inhibit the absorption of iron, while foods with calcium may reduce its bioavailability. Overall, when athletes eat a mixed diet including heme and nonheme iron sources, these inhibitory effects don't appear to negatively impact iron status. But because nonheme iron is less available, the RDA for vegetarians is 1.8 times higher than for those athletes who eat meat.[7]

As you can see in Table 3-1, iron requirements jump to 15 mg each day for the adolescent girl and 11 mg for the adolescent boy.[8] Female iron requirements are the highest, not only for growth and development, but also to cover menstrual losses. According to a 2012 survey called *What We Eat in America*, children aged 2 to 11 years consume 11.5 to 13.7 mg of iron each day, and teens aged 12 to 19 consume an average of 15.1 mg iron daily from food sources.[9] In athletes, however, low iron intake and iron deficiency are commonly reported.[10] A 2014 study showed higher rates of iron deficiency in female high school athletes aged 15 to 17; in that group, 52% had iron deficiency, and almost 9% had iron-deficiency anemia. Iron deficiency was present even for individuals with a higher iron intake and significantly less menstrual bleeding.[11]

When iron is deficient in the diet, low iron stores develop over time and can cause early fatigue, slow recovery from heavy–duty workouts, and a feeling of always being tired. Other symptoms of iron deficiency include stomach problems, decreased cognitive function, and disturbances in temperature regulation. Supplementation, managed by a medical professional, is generally required to correct iron deficiency.

Because Maggie had an established iron deficiency, her pediatrician started her on an iron supplement. Food alone would not have replenished her depleted iron stores. However, Maggie did need to eat more iron-rich foods so that once her blood iron returned to normal she could keep it there. Table 3-1 lists several iron-rich food sources.

Maggie was eating a mostly plant-based diet, so she also needed to understand the benefit of pairing vitamin C with iron-rich plant foods. This combination would increase her body's likelihood of absorbing the iron contained in plant foods. For example, Maggie loved spinach. Even though spinach is a high-iron source (3 mg iron in ½ cup [70 g]), she needed to add tomatoes or red peppers, which are rich in vitamin C, to a meal with spinach to increase its bioavailability. I also suggested she try beef or another meat once a week as a good source of iron and to optimize the absorption of the plant iron she was eating.

The Female Athlete Triad

Maggie had signs of the female athlete triad, a condition in which three characteristics coexist: low energy intake (with or without disordered eating), a lack of menstruation, and poor bone health. The female athlete triad is common in endurance athletes, such as long-distance runners. According to a 2013 study, as many as 16% of adolescent girls exhibit all three characteristics of the triad, and 50% to 60% demonstrate at least one or two of the three characteristics.[12] Girls with the triad have been noted to be osteopenic (exhibiting low bone density) and to have higher rates of stress fractures.[13] A more in-depth review of the triad is covered in Chapter 8.

Calcium and Vitamin D

Calcium and vitamin D are the bone-building nutrients. Bone building happens in the childhood and teen years and stops in early adulthood. In fact, 60% of adult cases of osteoporosis are related to low bone content developed during the teen years.[14] It's also thought that 20% of the variation in bone mass exhibited by individuals entering adulthood is due to variations in their earlier nutrition—including their intake of calcium and vitamin D—and the amount of weight-bearing exercise they did in their younger years.[15]

Calcium is a primary nutrient for bone health, but is also responsible for normal muscle contraction and blood clotting. It is tightly controlled in the body so that constant levels of calcium are maintained in the blood regardless of the consumption of calcium in food. In other words, the body will not let blood levels of calcium fluctuate based on food consumption. If dietary intake is inadequate, calcium will be pulled from the bones and delivered to the bloodstream.

To better understand this, think about a savings account at the bank. During the childhood and teen years, young athletes are making deposits into their savings account (bone). Once they reach adulthood, their bodies make withdrawals if not enough calcium is consumed, or the account remains steady if calcium intake is plentiful. In childhood and adolescence, the bone account grows, just like an investment account. Unfortunately, this isn't the case in adulthood—it's all about maintenance or depreciation.

As you can see in Table 3-1, from age 9 to 18 years, calcium needs jump to 1,300 mg per day, reflecting the peak bone-accumulation phase.[16] Research studies show that calcium intake is less than ideal in children and teens; more than 50% consume inadequate amounts. Girls are less likely to get the calcium they need than boys, and this holds true into adulthood.[17]

Although Maggie was referred to me for iron deficiency, an investigation of her overall diet told me she was not getting enough calcium and vitamin D. She did not like milk or yogurt and stayed away from cheese, and although she did eat lots of veggies, they just didn't add up to the amount of calcium she needed—1,300 mg a day. Young athletes who are most susceptible to calcium deficiency are those who avoid dairy products, are allergic to milk or soy, are vegetarian, or consume inadequate calories.[4,18]

Fortunately, there are many natural and fortified food sources of calcium, and children and teens tend to like many of them. Consistency is key for calcium intake, so you'll want to make sure it is part of your athlete's daily meal plan. Check out the best food sources of calcium in Table 3-1.

Even with fish as a mainstay, Maggie was also falling short on vitamin D, a fat-soluble vitamin that helps calcium be absorbed in the gut so it can enter the bones and be deposited. Vitamin D is also tied to the functionality and health of the immune system, and has a role in reducing inflammation.

An adequate vitamin D status comes from a diet rich in vitamin D and from exposure to direct sunlight, which enables vitamin D to be created in the skin. Even with these two sources available, meeting vitamin D needs can be challenging for the young athlete. According to a 2010 study in the *Clinical Journal of Sports Medicine*, 73% of athletes aged 14 to 17 years had insufficient vitamin D, as measured by their blood levels; the highest rates occurred among dancers, basketball players, and Tae Kwon Do competitors.[19] Not surprisingly, athletes who participated in indoor sports had higher rates of deficiency. Most children and teens do not experience physical symptoms of vitamin D deficiency until later in life. If you suspect your child has a vitamin D deficiency, discuss it with your health care provider and inquire about a blood test.

The well-established benefits of physical activity on bone health in kids and teens are traditionally connected to consuming enough calcium and dairy products. However, recent research has challenged this notion, showing that female athletes in high school who exercised for more than an hour a day and who had low vitamin D intake saw more stress fractures, regardless of calcium or dairy food intake.[20] The authors concluded that a higher vitamin D intake was predictive of a lower risk of developing stress fractures.

So where's the vitamin D? Vitamin D occurs naturally in a few foods—mainly salmon, tuna, and mackerel—and appears through fortification in others. Most vitamin D consumed in the American diet comes from fortified foods such as milk. Other dairy products, such as cheese and ice cream, are generally not fortified. Children and teens aged 1 to 18 require 600 international units (IU) per day.[21,22] Table 3-1 shows the best sources.

Athletes who can spend time outside in the sun and who consume foods rich in vitamin D are likely to have a sufficient vitamin D status. For young athletes who exercise indoors, live in high altitudes where sunshine may be limited to the warmer seasons, do not like dairy products or fish, or have dark skin pigmentation (which reduces vitamin D production in the skin), a vitamin D supplement may be beneficial.

Other Selected Micronutrients

All micronutrients are important, but often, when you focus on getting good amounts from food sources, other important micronutrients will fall into place. For example, when you focus on iron, zinc also goes up because iron and zinc are found together in foods such as beef, other meats, and beans. When you spend time working on getting more calcium in the diet, vitamin D is often increased as well because the two go hand in hand in many foods. When efforts are made to increase vitamin C, often vitamin A rises as well because both are found in many fruits and vegetables. The easiest ways to make sure your young athletes get all their micronutrients each day is for them to eat a balanced diet that includes a wide variety of different food, while targeting the recommended daily servings for each food group, something I'll cover in more detail in Chapter 5.

Let's briefly explore some of the other micronutrients that are important to your athlete's health and wellness, and don't forget to check the RDA, UL, and food sources in Table 3-1.

Vitamin B Complex. The B complex vitamins include thiamin (B_1), riboflavin (B_2), niacin, pyridoxine (B_6), pantothenic acid, biotin, folate, and vitamin B_{12}. The main role of these water-soluble vitamins is to make sure that energy is produced in the body's cells, and that muscle is built and repaired. Folate and vitamin B_{12} are the B vitamins that play a role in red blood cell production, protein creation, and tissue repair. Some research has suggested that exercise creates a greater need for B complex vitamins, up to twice the RDA,[23] though most experts agree that an increased need for B vitamins can be met by simply increasing the calorie intake in the diet. Young athletes who are vegetarian or who have disordered eating patterns, including tight calorie control of food intake or skipping meals, are at the highest risk for low intake of riboflavin, B_6, folate, and B_{12}. Deficiency of B vitamins may worsen performance during high-intensity exercise and may reduce the ability to repair and build muscle. Severe deficiency of folate or vitamin B_{12} may cause anemia, which can curtail exercise endurance.

Vitamin C. Citrus fruits and many vegetables naturally provide vitamin C, an important water-soluble vitamin involved in immunity and healing.

It also plays a role in helping the body absorb non-heme iron, as discussed on page 72. Most children and teens meet their daily requirement for vitamin C.

Vitamin A. Vitamin A is a fat-soluble vitamin that helps with vision and the immune system. Most children and teens consume enough vitamin A in their diet, although this decreases with age, especially in girls and African-American children.[24]

Vitamin E. As an antioxidant, vitamin E helps get rid of cell-damaging free radicals, which can cause heart disease and cancer. It also plays a role in immunity.

Zinc. Zinc is involved in many functions in the body, including immunity, growth, wound healing, and proper taste and smell. In athletes, a zinc deficiency can cause loss of appetite, weight loss, fatigue, and lowered endurance.[25]

Selenium. Selenium plays a key role in reproduction, thyroid regulation, and immunity, and acts as an antioxidant.

Magnesium. Magnesium is involved in many metabolic reactions in the body, including energy metabolism, blood sugar control, blood pressure regulation, protein creation, and muscle function. Dietary surveys show that magnesium intake is low, especially among teenage girls.[26] Foods containing dietary fiber are good sources of magnesium.

Eating a Well-Balanced Diet

Whether or not you meet your daily requirements for micronutrients relies upon what you're eating, how much, and how frequently—in other words, the variety and balance in your diet. With over 40 nutrients to address in the growing athlete's diet, I don't expect you to keep track of your child's every little morsel and micronutrient. The key to success is planning a well-balanced diet. I'll tell you how in Chapter 5.

While eating a variety of foods every day is important, making sure your athlete's diet is made up of mostly whole, natural foods (such as fresh fruit, veggies, whole grains, lean protein, low-fat dairy, and healthy fats) is also critical. Unfortunately, many of the foods kids and teens like to eat are full of calories and fat but are lacking in nutrients. A nutrient-poor, calorie-rich diet means your growing athlete may have to work harder at his or her sport.

Although popular opinion would suggest that all packaged and processed foods are bad, fortunately this is not the case. Many convenience foods like cereal, bread products, orange juice, and granola bars have been fortified with added vitamins and minerals, making them a nutrient-rich option for kids and teens alike. For instance, ready-to-eat cereals and breads are often fortified with calcium, iron, and folic acid, making them a nutritious choice at mealtime. While there will always be drawbacks, such as too much sugar in breakfast cereal, you will be better able to match micronutrient needs when you know what to look for on an ingredients label (see box).

Making Sense of Ingredients Label Daily Values

The U.S. Food and Drug Administration (FDA) developed Daily Values (DVs) to help people read food labels and be able to recognize good sources of nutrients. Each nutrient has a DV—for example, for iron, the DV is 18 mg, and for vitamin D, it is 400 IU. Foods that provide 20% or more of the DV are considered to be high sources of a nutrient. Foods that rank lower, such as 5% DV, aren't considered good sources, but they can add value to your athlete's diet. The DV is particularly helpful if you are targeting specific nutrients in the diet.

The good news is that your athlete *can* meet all the requirements for vitamins and minerals with a balanced diet representing a variety of food. The bad news is this reality: getting your athlete to eat balanced meals day in and day out is hard. It requires planning ahead, a dedication to cooking, and a young athlete with a cooperative palate. For some athletes, the busy-ness of life, their individual food preferences, and their daily eating habits will make the use of a vitamin and mineral supplement beneficial.

The Pros and Cons of Vitamin and Mineral Supplements

Used as an insurance policy to cover gaps in nutrition, micronutrient supplementation is one of the most common "fix-it" strategies for the modern diet, and athletes are not immune to jumping on this bandwagon. Lately, the belief that these micronutrients can enhance athletic performance has become popular. A 2005 survey in the United Kingdom found that 62% of teens were using supplements, mostly of vitamins and minerals, in order to improve health, immune function, and performance.[27] In a 2012 United States study, about 1.2 million children and teens (1.6% of estimated youth sports participants) reported using some type of supplement to enhance sports performance. Of this group, 94% used multivitamin and mineral combination supplements, fiber, and/or fish oil specifically to enhance sports performance.[28] However, there is no evidence that suggests better sports performance in children and teens when vitamins, minerals, or other nutrients are added.

In general, pinpointing one vitamin or mineral and supplementing it is not advised unless a true deficient state has been established, as with Maggie and her iron deficiency. When a deficiency has been identified, usually by blood tests, a medical professional will be able to correct it with a nutrient supplement. This is a reasonable expectation for iron, B_{12}, and folate deficiencies.

One thing that is often overlooked in assessing whether an athlete needs a supplement is the intake of fortified foods. As I mentioned above, many food products are fortified, such as cereal, yogurt, bread, and pasta, which is a good thing because fortification has historically reversed some devastating deficiencies; for example, we guard against neural tube defects (spina bifida) with folic acid fortification of foods. However, when fortified foods are combined with a vitamin and mineral supplement, the young athlete can enter into dangerous territory and micronutrient toxicity can result. In this scenario, vitamin A and folic acid are at greatest concern for toxicity.

I like to look at each individual athlete—his or her diet, exercise, and growth phase—before recommending a supplement. I always suggest modifying food intake, even as a complement to a prescribed nutrient supplement, such as iron. I tend to steer away from anything more than the standard RDA dose, and am wary of claims or promises that suggest improved athleticism or performance. Safety and adequacy are always my first concerns. I hope you adopt this discretion too. Always check with your doctor or nutrition professional to see if a supplement is warranted, and to determine a safe dosage.

Six Signs that Your Young Athlete May Need a Nutrient Supplement

Some young athletes may need a vitamin and mineral supplement, despite your best efforts at healthy nutrition. Young athletes may need supplementation if they do any of the following:

1. They avoid one or more food groups: An absence or lack of fruits, vegetables, protein, dairy, or grains can translate to low intakes of vitamins (A, C, D, and the B complex), potassium, calcium, and other micronutrients.
2. They consume high amounts of calorie-rich, nutrient-poor snack foods: Eating too many unhealthy snacks may mean young athletes are missing out on a variety of micronutrients.
3. They consume low amounts of meat and beans: Iron, zinc, and vitamin B_{12} may be of concern.
4. They have a low body weight: Low calorie intake may translate to low nutrient intake.
5. They are careful or selective eaters: Young athletes who limit their eating and are particular about food may not be getting enough nutrients, especially iron, calcium, and vitamin D. A multivitamin and mineral supplement with iron may be beneficial, as well as a calcium supplement (vitamin and mineral supplements typically contain very low amounts of calcium).
6. They skip dairy foods and nondairy substitutions: Calcium and vitamin D will be the losers in this scenario, so a supplemental

calcium and vitamin D chew or tablet may be needed. Check with your health care provider.

While I don't expect you to become an expert on micronutrients, I do believe that the more you know, the better able you will be to keep your athlete nourished and healthy. When so much attention is given to the starting lineup (macronutrients), you may be forgetting about some important vitamins and minerals that will surely impact your athlete's performance and overall health. Knowing where and how to balance micronutrients will help prevent adverse health and performance outcomes. Showcasing a variety of high-nutrient foods, in the right amount, will only help your athlete stay healthy and perform at his or her best.

Notes

1. Food and Nutrition Board, Institute of Medicine, National Academies. "Dietary Reference Intakes for vitamin A, vitamin K, arsenic, boron, chromium, copper, iodine, iron, manganese, molybdenum, nickel, silicon, vanadium, and zinc" (2001); and "Dietary reference intakes for calcium and vitamin D" (2011). www.nap.edu.
2. National Institutes of Health. Office of Dietary Supplements. "Vitamin B_6." http://ods.od.nih.gov/factsheets/VitaminB6-HealthProfessional/.
3. Jeukendrup A and Cronin L. "Nutrition and elite young athletes." *Med Sport Sci.* 56 (2011): 47–58.
4. U.S. Department of Agriculture and U.S. Department of Health and Human Services. "*Dietary Guidelines for Americans, 2015.*" Available at: http://www.health.gov/dietaryguidelines/2015-scientific-report/PDFs/Scientific-Report-of-the-2015-Dietary-Guidelines-Advisory-Committee.pdf
5. Meyer F, O'Connor H, Shirreffs SM, and the International Association of Athletics Federations. "Nutrition for the young athlete." *J Sports Sci.* 25 (2007): S73–S82.
6. Evans MW, Ndetan H, Perko M, Williams R, and Walker C. "Dietary supplement use by children and adolescents in the United States to enhance sport performance. Results of the National Health Interview Study." *J Prim Prev.* 33 (2012): 3–12.

7. National Institutes of Health. Office of Dietary Supplements. "Iron." http:// ods.od.nih.gov/factsheets/Iron-HealthProfessional/.

8. Food and Nutrition Board, Institute of Medicine, National Academies, op. cit.

9. U.S. Department of Agriculture. Agricultural Research Service. What We Eat in America, 2009–2010. http://www.ars.usda.gov/SP2UserFiles/Place/ 80400530/pdf/0910/tables_1-40_2009-2010.pdf.

10. Meyer et al, op. cit.

11. Sandstrom G, Borjesson M, and Rodjer S. "Iron deficiency in adolescent female athletes—is iron status affected by regular sporting activity?" *Clin J Sports Med*. 22 (2012): 495–500.

12. Barrack MT, Ackerman KE, and Gibbs JC. "Update on the female athlete triad." *Curr Rev Musculoskelet Med*. 6 (2013): 195–204.

13. Ibid.

14. Valtuena J, Gracia-Marco L, Vicente-Rodriguez G, Gonzalez-Gross M, Huybrechts I, Rey-Lopez JP, Mouratidou T, Sioen I, Mesana MI, Martinez AE, Widhalm K, Moreno LA, and the HELENA study group. "Vitamin D status and physical activity interact to improve bone mass in adolescents. The HELENA study." *Osteoporosis Int*. 23 (2012): 2227–2237.

15. Ibid.

16. Food and Nutrition Board, Institute of Medicine, National Academies, op. cit.

17. Marriott BP, Olsho L, Hadden L, and Connor P. "Intake of added sugars and selected nutrients in the United States, National Health and Nutrition Examination Survey (NHANES) 2003–2006." *Crit Rev Food Sci Nutr*. 50 (2010): 228–258.

18. U.S. Department of Agriculture, Agricultural Research Service. 2014. USDA National Nutrient Database for Standard Reference, Release 27. Nutrient Data Laboratory home page. http://www.ars.usda.gov/ba/bhnrc/ ndl.

19. Constantini NW, Arieli R, CHodick G, and Dubnov-Raz G. "High prevalence of vitamin D insufficiency in athletes and dancers." *Clin J Sports Med*. 20 (2010): 368–371.

20. Sonneville KR, Gordon CM, and Field AE. "Vitamin D, calcium, and dairy intakes and stress fractures among female adolescents." *Arch Pediatr Adolesc Med*. 166 (2012): 595–600.

21. Food and Nutrition Board, Institute of Medicine, National Academies, op. cit.

22. U.S. Department of Agriculture, Agricultural Research Service, op. cit.

23. Woolf K and Manore MM. "B-vitamins and exercise: does exercise alter requirements?" *Int J Sport Nutr Exerc Metab.* 16 (2006): 453–484.
24. National Institutes of Health. Office of Dietary Supplements. "Vitamin A." http://ods.od.nih.gov/factsheets/VitaminA-HealthProfessional/.
25. Micheletti A, Rossi R, and Rufini S. "Zinc status in athletes. Relation to diet and exercise." *Sports Med.* 31 (2001): 577–582.
26. National Institutes of Health. Office of Dietary Supplements. "Magnesium." http://ods.od.nih.gov/factsheets/Magnesium-HealthProfessional/.
27. Petroczi A, Naughton DP, Mazanov J, Holloway A, and Bingham J. "Limited agreement exists between rationale and practice in athletes' supplement use for maintenance of health: a retrospective study." *Nutr J.* 6 (2007): 34.
28. Evans et al, op. cit.

CHAPTER 4

The Relief Pitcher:
Fluids and Hydration

*If you don't eat right as an athlete, you'll get tired and won't be as sharp.
It's simple to drink sodas and sports drinks, but water is the most essential
drink to put in your body.*
—Troy Polamalu, strong safety, Pittsburgh Steelers

Julie was a three-sport athlete, but spring track was her
favorite; she had always done well and had advanced to the
state finals for 2 years in a row. As a 17-year-old junior, she
knew the routine: practice every day after school, log good
weekend mileage, and compete in track meets during the
week. She thought her nutrition plan was adequate—she ate
three meals and snacked on apples, peanut butter, yogurt,
and granola—but her biggest challenge was drinking. "To be
honest, I am lazy when it comes to tracking my fluid intake,"
said Julie. "I'd rather be talking with my friends instead of
going to the water fountain or through the lunch line to buy a
drink." By midseason, she had started to experience cramping,
nausea, and terrible headaches after workouts, and came to
me after her pediatrician diagnosed her with dehydration.
What Julie needed was a hydration plan she could execute
consistently.

One of the fastest ways for an athlete to tank his or her performance is to become dehydrated. Julie clearly wasn't drinking enough after running, nor was she loading up during the day in preparation for her practice. As a result, she was experiencing subtle side effects in her performance: thinking she was hungry after practice when she was really thirsty, and suffering from stomach cramps midway through practices. Once Julie started a foolproof hydration plan and monitored her urine, it was easier for her to stay hydrated.

Unfortunately, many growing children and teen athletes like Julie don't pay attention to how much they drink throughout the day. They wait to drink until they're thirsty (which may be too late) and get behind on their daily fluid intake. According to University of South Carolina athletic training professor Dr. Susan Yearning, up to 75% of athletes aged 8 to 18 come to practice dehydrated.[1] Kids, parents, and coaches need to know about dehydration and its signs and symptoms, as well as how to prevent it. But before dehydration can be fully understood, you need to know how much fluid the body needs under normal, non-exercising conditions. The amount of fluids your body requires to maintain a normal hydration status is called your *daily fluid needs*.

There are three easy ways for your young athlete to meet his or her daily fluid needs:

- *Drink 1 milliliter (mL) of fluid for every calorie the body requires.*[2] For example, if your 10-year-old, moderately active boy needs 1,900 calories, he needs to drink 1,900 milliliters of fluid (there are 30 mL in 1 ounce of fluid, so he would need 63 ounces, or 8 cups a day). Basic calorie requirements for your child or teen appear in Chapter 1.
- *Use the weight rule.*[3] Kids who weigh over 44 pounds (20 kg) need 1,500 milliliters plus 10 milliliters per pound for each pound over 44 pounds (20 kg). So your 55-pound (25-kg) 9-year-old needs about 1,610 milliliters (54 ounces or 6½ cups) per day. Kids over 66 pounds (30 kg) need 1,700 milliliters plus 5 milliliters per pound for each pound over 66 pounds (30 kg). A 112-pound (51-kg) freshman requires 1,930 milliliters (64 ounces or 8 cups) per day.
- *Use the population standards called the Dietary Reference Intake (DRI).*[4] Eight-year-olds need 7 cups (1.66 L) per day; 9- to 13-year-old boys need 10 cups (2.37 L) per day; 9- to 13-year-old girls need 7 to

8 cups (1.66 to 1.9 L) per day; 14- to 18-year-old boys need 13 cups (3.1 L) per day; 14-to 18-year-old girls need 9 to 10 cups (2.13 to 2.37 L) per day.

Most healthy children and teens drink enough fluids to meet their everyday needs, especially if their meals and snacks include a variety of fluids. Other foods like fruit, veggies, soup, and yogurt provide fluid too, so the burden doesn't solely rest on liquids. When it comes to the way the body handles fluid—how it is distributed throughout the cells, muscle, and organs, and how hormones fine-tune the balance—there is little difference between children and adults, despite a significant difference in body size.[5] The small difference that exists lies in children's drinking behaviors—what they choose, when they drink, and how much. I'll discuss this later in the chapter.

Thermoregulation: Keeping Your Body's AC Running

Thermoregulation is a fancy word for your body's air conditioning system. It's the ability to adjust internal body heat, whether under extreme temperatures, like exercising outside in Tampa during the month of August, or just staying cool on a hot summer's day. Not too long ago, it was thought that children weren't able to adjust and control their internal body temperature as well as adults, placing them at a higher risk for dehydration. However, recent studies that directly compare adults with children have shown that children are equally good at thermoregulation, even in hot, humid conditions.[6]

Sweating is an obvious, unavoidable by-product of exercise, and an important one. Sweating is the way the body releases heat that builds up inside. It allows the rising internal heat to exit the body, cooling the skin and lowering the internal heat index. If you weren't able to sweat, your internal body temperature would increase to dangerous levels—in essence, cooking your insides and damaging your internal organs. It's not only fluids that are released from the body when you sweat; sodium, chloride, and potassium also leave. These substances—called electrolytes—

help muscles contract and function well, so it's important to replace them during and after exercise. Plenty of fluid, scheduled breaks, and proper clothing go a long way to regulate the effects of sweating too much or too little.

Everyone has a different sweat profile, releasing higher or lower amounts of electrolytes and rates of sweating. Some people are heavy sweaters and may be prone to dehydration, while others barely sweat at all and may be prone to overheating. Sam was a heavy sweater. As a 14-year-old junior rower, he spent many days on the ergometer (rowing machine) working out. When he took his workouts outside during the summer, he noticed big salt rings around his neck and armpits when he was done. This was an indication that he was losing large amounts of salt in his sweat and needed to replace it with a salt-containing beverage, like Gatorade, or salty foods (pretzels or crackers) paired with water.

Rates of sweating depend on individual characteristics, as well as the clothing worn, the environmental temperature, the intensity of the activity, and one's overall hydration status. And of course, during heavy exercise the body sweats more. Pay attention to how much your young athletes sweat, as it provides key information to help you hydrate them and prevent dehydration.

When it comes to kids and sweating, there are differences based on sex and the stage of puberty. Children generally have lower sweat rates than teens and adults. The average sweat rate for boys and girls aged 11 to 14 years old is about 2 to 4 cups (474 to 948 mL) per hour during exercise, according to a 2007 study.[7] Boys sweat less than men, but once puberty hits, sweat rates become comparable to those of adult men. In contrast, girls have similar rates of sweating to those of women, regardless of the stage of puberty they're in.

The Dangers of Dehydration

Every year around the start of school (when the heat of the summer hasn't abated), we hear tragic stories involving young athletes who have suffered from heat illness, heat stroke, and even death as a result of dehydration. The high school football player who, in full pads, collapses on the

field; the track athlete who is disoriented, stumbles, and barely crosses the finish line; and the lacrosse player who suffers heat stroke and needs an ice down—these stories are becoming more common across the United States.

Did you know that heat stroke is the third-highest exercise-related cause of death in high school students?[8] Heat illness, heat stroke, and death are preventable, which makes stories like these even more disturbing.

The two main reasons for dehydration are low fluid intake and too much sweating. While we cannot change our biological sweating tendencies, we can alter how we dress and how much we drink to reduce our chances of becoming dehydrated. Thankfully, today's young athletes have plenty of climate- sensitive clothing available to them, making it easier for them to stay cool and dry.

Kids and teens don't get dehydrated on purpose. As a parent, dietitian, and even volunteer coach at one time, I've seen kids forget water bottles, not take the time to drink, and get distracted from rehydrating. While this is completely typical of kids of all ages, the outcome can be serious. Coaches and parents need to be vigilant, not just reminding kids to drink but actually making sure they do.

One way to help your young athlete understand the importance of hydration is to compare muscles to either raisins or to grapes, depending on how much and how often your athlete drinks. *Dehydrated* muscles are like raisins—dry, stiff, and shriveled—and, as such, they lose their ability to react quickly, and possibly get stuck in a contracted state, also known as a muscle cramp. *Hydrated* muscles are like grapes—soft, supple, and plump—and, as such, they contain the right amount of water and salt to perform normally. Athletes want grapes, not raisins, for the best athletic performance.

When Heat Stroke Strikes, Act Fast!

If your young athlete shows signs of unusual fatigue, confusion, headache, muscle cramps, nausea, vomiting, lack of sweating, racing heartbeat, rapid and shallow breathing, or flushed skin, you may have a case of heat stroke on your hands. According to the Mayo Clinic guidelines for treating heat stroke, you'll want to bring down the athlete's

core body temperature as soon as possible, using any of the following measures: place cold, wet towels in the corners of the groin and
armpits, and around the neck and head; submerge the athlete in an
ice bath; blow a fan directly on the athlete; and call 911 for medical
assistance.[9]

A phenomenon called *voluntary dehydration* may increase the risk for
dehydration. It occurs when kids and teens are no longer thirsty because
they have been drinking, but have not consumed enough to make them
fully hydrated. Consider the young basketball player who, during a time-
out, takes one swig of water, then heads back onto the court. One swig
is roughly 1 ounce (30 mL)—maybe enough to quench his thirst for the
time being, but not enough to hydrate him. Add up these individual gulps
over the course of a game, and this athlete still will likely fall short on
hydration. Children are at the highest risk for voluntary dehydration, as
are those who have exercised in hot, humid conditions.[10]

Dehydration progresses along a continuum, beginning with mild dehydration and progressing to severe dehydration, and is outlined in Table
4-1. When young athletes become progressively dehydrated, their symptoms become more severe. Their bodies become less able to sweat and thus
adjust their internal thermometer, so the body temperature rises. Their
brain becomes confused, and their decision making becomes hampered.
The heart needs to work harder to pump blood throughout the body, causing the pulse to increase and the breathing to become more rapid. Plus,
the functioning of their muscles becomes compromised and they may
perform less well.

A classic sign of dehydration is weight loss. Even a small amount of
weight loss due to dehydration can curtail athletic performance, as in the
case of mild dehydration. One study looked at 10- to 12-year-old boys
with as little as 1% dehydration (about ½ to 1 pound [0.23 to 0.45 kg] of
weight loss after exercise) and showed that their exercise endurance was
shortened.[11] It's different for teens and adults, whose athletic function may
remain intact with up to a 2% dehydration level (up to 2 pounds [0.9 kg]
of weight loss in a 100-pound [45-kg] athlete). Table 4-1 looks at weight
loss and the potential signs and symptoms of dehydration.

Table 4-1 Signs and Symptoms of Dehydration in Children and Teens

Dehydration Level	Weight Loss (Post-Exercise) in the Athlete Weighing . . .				Signs	Performance Outcome
	60 lb	80 lb	100 lb	150 lb		
1–2% (mild)	½ to 1 lb weight loss	¾ to 1½ lb weight loss	1 to 2 lb weight loss	1½ to 3 lb weight loss	Thirsty, restless, dry mouth, fatigue, headache	Decreased endurance, alertness, and cognitive function
3–4% (mild to moderate)	1¾ to 2½ lb weight loss	2½ to 3¼ lb weight loss	3 to 4 lb weight loss	4½ to 6 lb weight loss	Reduced sweating, headache, increased thirst, fatigue, cramping	Decline in athletic performance; confusion
5–9% (moderate)	3 to 5½ lb weight loss	4 to 7¼ lb weight loss	5 to 9 lb weight loss	7½ to 13½ lb weight loss	Lethargic, drowsy, dizzy, irritability, muscle cramps	Above plus decreased performance in distance events
> 10% (severe)	> 6 lb weight loss	> 8 lb weight loss	> 10 lb weight loss	> 12 lb weight loss	Apprehensive, cold, blue extremities, muscle cramps, seizures, cardiac arrest	Above plus decreased sweat production, blood flow, and cardiac output

Some athletes use dehydration techniques to lose weight in a short period of time, relying on dangerous tricks like wearing a rubber suit while working out, turning up the heat in the gym, taking diuretics, or even fasting. For quick weight loss, some athletes vomit, induce diarrhea, or stop eating and drinking the day before or day of competition.

Why the crazy weight-loss schemes? Some sports are organized by weight class and require a weigh-in before a competition to make sure athletes meet particular weight standards. If athletes don't make the weight cut, they won't be able to compete. Rowing, wrestling, boxing, various martial arts, and horseback riding are some of the sports that require a weigh-in before competition is allowed.

When young athletes embark on quick weight loss through dehydration and simultaneous overtraining, a condition called *rhabdomyolysis* can occur in which muscle tissue breaks down, overloading the body with a massive release of broken-down muscle fibers. These products overload the kidneys and heart, and may cause kidney failure, heart malfunction, and even death.

Drastic efforts to lose weight are not recommended for growing children and teens, and they may increase the risk for disordered eating, self-starvation, and other adverse medical conditions.

Hydrate for Health

The easiest way to ensure that your athlete is drinking enough is to have a drinking plan, one that covers daily fluid needs plus extra to cover exercise. A good drinking plan is laid out in three phases: before, during, and after exercise.

To kick things off on the right foot, make sure that before exercise your young athletes are already hydrated—this means drinking throughout the day. Second, make sure they are drinking during exercise, which means that they have packed enough fluids or have access to them during exercise. Finally, make sure they have a plan to recover with fluids once exercise is completed—the after-exercise drinking. All this drinking helps the body remain in prime form and replenishes fluids lost during sweating and exercise. It has the added benefit of preventing subsequent dehydration, which may compound symptoms and side effects for future competitions. It's easy for athletes who don't have a drinking plan to become dehydrated.

To help keep your athletes on track, review their daily fluid intake (when and how much); remind them to keep fluids close at hand; ask them to drink at every break during exercise, taking at least three or four gulps (3 to 4 ounces [90 to 120 mL] at a time; and warn them to never let their sports bottle stay empty.

Nudging athletes with reminders may do the trick for some of them, but others like to have specific guidelines for their drinking plan. Here's what the scientists say (if you want a practical translation, check out Table 4-2):

- *Before exercise*: Drink 6 milliliters per pound of body weight per hour (a 100-pound [45-kg] athlete needs 600 mL, or about 20 oz, per hour) 2 to 3 hours before exercise.[12]
- *During exercise*: Drink about 20 ounces (600 mL) per hour, the equivalent of 4 ounces (½ cup [120 mL]), every 10 to 15 minutes.[13]
- *After exercise*: Nine- to 12-year-old children should replenish with 3 to 8 ounces (90 to 237 mL) of fluid every 20 minutes, and adolescents may consume 32 to 48 ounces (948 to 1,422 mL) of fluid every hour, until hydrated, according to the American Academy of Pediatrics (AAP).[14] Or drink 2 milliliters per pound of body weight per hour (a 100-pound [45-kg] child needs 200 mL per hour, or about 7 oz), within 1 to 2 hours after exercise.

Once your athlete feels thirsty, he or she may already be dehydrated. According to the Institute of Medicine and other prominent researchers, a young athlete can use thirst as a gauge for knowing when and how much fluid to drink. This is partly due to studies showing that young athletes voluntarily drink enough during exercise—about 75% of their sweat volume, leaving only a slight body water deficit to be addressed at the end of exercise.[15]

The "drink when you're thirsty" advice, though, relies on ready access to fluids and an accurate perception of thirst. Each athlete has an individualized perception of thirst, and taste preferences can influence that perception. Some young athletes will hold out for what they *like* to drink,

Table 4-2 When and How Much to Drink

Weight of Athlete	Before Exercise (2 to 3 hours prior)	During Exercise (Every 15 minutes)	After Exercise (Drink every hour for 1 to 2 hours beyond normal drinking volume)
60 lb	¾ cup (177 mL)	3 ounces (85 mL)	½ cup (118 mL)
80 lb	2 cups (473 mL)	½ cup (119 mL)	¾ cup (177 mL)
100 lb	2½ cups (591 mL)	⅔ cup (159 mL)	¾ to 1 cup (177 to 237 mL)
120 lb	3 cups (710 mL)	¾ cup (177 mL)	1 cup (237 mL)
150 lb	3¾ cups (887 mL)	~1 cup (237 mL)	1¼ cup (296 mL)

rather than what they *need* to drink. Others find it hard to make the time they need for drinking and become used to not drinking during exercise, a habit that may translate to a perception of not being thirsty. In addition, if athletes aren't acclimated to a hot and humid climate (for example, if there's a heat wave in May), their perception of thirst may be off.

Unlike adult athletes, who are better at self-regulating their hydration, children need adult guidance. Dr. Thomas Rowland, pediatric cardiologist at the Baystate Medical Center in Springfield, Massachusetts, says, "Kids will drink enough by thirst, but because they're immature and easily distracted, coaches need to take responsibility for regular fluid replacement breaks to keep their attention on keeping hydrated."

I've seen too many young athletes become distracted by their surroundings; they don't know how important it is to hydrate, they don't have a sense of when to drink, and they even ignore thirst, so a more formalized approach is needed. "The difference between child and adult athletes is really a matter of who's taking responsibility for keeping [them] hydrated," emphasizes Rowland.

Recent research throws the thirst perception advice into question. A 2013 study looked at 107 boys aged 11 to 16 who were attending a summer soccer camp. Most of the boys were underhydrated before practice, meaning they had a body water deficit before starting exercise. Researchers monitored their hydration status during two subsequent days of soccer training and found the boys continued to be dehydrated, at increasing rates; 96% were dehydrated on day 2 and 97% were dehydrated on day 3, despite having easy access to plenty of water. The authors concluded that drinking according to thirst may not be sufficient for young athletes, and that coaches, trainers, and other athletes need to constantly make an effort to enhance hydration in young athletes.[16]

What Is Over-Hydration?

Also called water intoxication, over-hydration happens when young athletes over-drink fluids (more than the body is able to urinate), resulting in dangerously low amounts of sodium in the blood. The symptoms of over-hydration include bloating, pale urine, swelling of hands and feet, throbbing headache, and rapid weight gain. Advanced signs include digestive problems, such as nausea and vomiting; seizure; and coma. The brain is the most susceptible body organ to over-hydration.

Helping your young athletes make sure they drink enough can be difficult, but taking the time to outline a basic drinking plan with them is worth the effort. Such a plan offers a reference point and underlines the importance of hydration. Some young athletes do better at staying hydrated when their beverages are flavored, so make sure to find the best approach for your child or teen.[17] The drinking plan will likely change each year as your young athlete grows and stabilizes closer to adulthood. Use Table 4-2 to gauge amounts and timing for hydration.

Double-Check Your Young Athlete's Hydration Status

Even when you follow guidelines for how much your young athlete drinks every day, it's important to make sure he or she is getting enough fluids. There are easy ways to monitor hydration status.

Weight Checks

Checking weight is a way to figure out an athlete's sweat rate—how much water is lost through sweating.[18] Here's how to do it: Weigh your athlete before exercise (after using the bathroom, wearing minimal clothing) and then again after exercise. The total body weight lost reflects the amount of fluid that is lost through sweating. *Rule of thumb*: for every pound lost, the young athlete should drink about 2 cups (474 mL) of fluid.

Thirst

You can estimate thirst level by using a number scale, where 1 is not thirsty at all and 9 is very, very thirsty. If your child or teen falls between 3 (a little thirsty) and 5 (moderately thirsty), it's fair to assume he or she is mildly dehydrated (a 1% to 2% body weight deficit signifying mild to moderate dehydration).[19]

Urine Color

Urine color is another easy way to determine whether your athlete is hydrated or dehydrated. Young athletes need to have a urine color that is very pale yellow, like fresh-squeezed lemonade. Golden yellow, medium yellow, orangey, or brownish-green urine are all signs of dehydration. The darker the color of the urine, the more dehydrated the athlete.[20]

What to Drink: The Beverages of Choice

If I could wave my magic dietitian wand and cast a spell, making all young athletes drink a magic potion to help them perform at their peak, I would. But what would that magic potion be? Ideally, water first, then a sports drink *during* an extended exercise session.

When athletes are not exercising, I'd want them to drink water, three servings of milk or a nondairy alternative like soymilk each day, and maybe a small amount of 100% juice. No soda, no energy drinks, and no sugary juices.

However, I am not Glenda the Good Witch, nor do I have the ability to make each athlete drink the healthiest beverages on the planet. And the reality is, sugary drinks are going to slip in here and there. Nevertheless, you do have enormous influence in keeping your athlete's drink choices healthy and effective.

According to the 2015 Dietary Guidelines for Americans (DGA), children and teens consume a significant amount of calories per day from beverages including milk, regular soda, energy and sports drinks, fruit drinks, and 100% fruit juice. Children consume more milk and 100% fruit juice (that's good), and teens consume more soda (that's bad).[21] Unfortunately, we see more and more of the teen drinking trends infiltrating athletic fields and courts, chipping away at the health quality of the young athlete's diet.

If given free reign, children and teens tend to choose food and beverages based on their taste preferences.[22] However, they may not understand that relying on tasty drinks can backfire, resulting in poor nutrient intake, unneeded calories, and even potentially dangerous substances. Don't be fooled into thinking your young athlete is making good decisions about what to drink. I see plenty of athletes drinking soda, giant bottles of juice, and—worse—energy shots.

How do you reduce your young athletes' intake of sugary drinks and other undesirable beverages? Let's look at the options young athletes have and investigate their pros and cons so that you can advise them on the best options.

Water

Our bodies are made up of many cells, and those cells are filled with water. So common sense would tell us that drinking water is essential—and it is. Plain water should be the mainstay of an athlete's fluid diet—on and off the court, all day, every day. Plain old water trumps juice boxes and sports drinks for the under-13 crowd, because games and practices for that age group are typically under an hour. In fact, water is the best fluid to use while exercising for less than 1 hour and may be totally fine in longer exercise sessions for some athletes.[23] Water is absorbed easily, tolerated well, and portable. Cool or cold water is most acceptable, so lug along the cooler or ice-down the water bottle.

On today's sports scene, you'll also find "enhanced" and "fitness" waters like those from Propel, VitaminWater, or SmartWater. These may contain anything from added antioxidants and vitamins to natural and artificial flavors and sugars. In general, they don't provide enough carbohydrate for the exercising athlete, so athletes shouldn't use them during long sessions (over an hour). While they are okay for a short workout and the flavored versions may be better accepted taste-wise, buyer beware—those extra vitamins and antioxidants aren't scientifically proven to enhance anything, except maybe the hole in your wallet.

Another category of water is marketed as "premium hydration."[24] These waters and beverages—products such as alkaline waters, electrolyte-enhanced waters and beverages, naturally functional products such as coffee- and fruit-based drinks, and any number of coconut waters—promise natural refreshment, improved function, and a tasty alternative to plain water. The problem is that premium water comes at a premium price but with no proof of premium performance.

Sports Drinks

Sports drinks were designed to ward off fatigue and prevent athletes from becoming dehydrated. Yet many Americans, young and old, use them, whether they are athletes or not. Traditional sports drinks such as Gatorade and Powerade offer carbohydrate as an energy source, and sodium, potassium, and chloride to help replenish the loss of electrolytes in sweat.

One unique element of sports drinks is the carbohydrate source. Various sugars, such as fructose, sucrose, and dextrose, are included, so muscles can use different carbohydrate absorption pathways, promoting the best muscular performance. You won't find this unique benefit in fruit juices or soda. The total amount of carbohydrate in sports drinks ranges from 14 to 19 grams in a 1-cup (237 mL) serving size. Young athletes using sports drinks containing higher amounts (16–18 g) of carbohydrate have been shown to experience stomach cramps, so a lower total sugar content may be better tolerated.[25]

Newer sports-drink products (for example, Powerade + B vitamins) offer B vitamins and claim to enhance performance, although there is no convincing evidence of this. Unless a vitamin B deficiency exists, which is rare, the B vitamins in these sports drinks simply end up in the toilets of most athletes.

The most important thing to remember is that sports drinks are appropriate only for child and teen athletes exercising in hot weather, participating in exercise lasting longer than an hour, or engaging in multiple exercise sessions per day. Sports drinks are popular among all kids and teens, and their "health halo"—the idea that they are healthy—is part of the reason. More than a quarter of parents (27%) believe sports drinks are healthy beverages for their children.[26] As a result, the overall consumption of sports drinks is increasing. One study of children aged 6 to 11 years showed a sixfold increase (from 2% to 12%) in consumption rates from 1989 to 2008, while total amounts consumed also increased from about 8 ounces (237 mL) per day to almost 10 ounces (296 mL) per day.[27]

The Over/Under Rule for Sports Drinks

Over an hour. Choose a sports drink to provide your young athlete's body with a source of carbohydrate, salt, and potassium, and drink enough to stay hydrated.

Under an hour. Choose water. Kids aren't burning enough calories or sweating enough to warrant using anything else.

One of the side effects of overusing sports drinks is extra weight gain. In a 2012 study, children and teens aged 9 to 15 saw an average weight gain of 3.5 pounds (1.6 kg) per year (or a 0.3 increase in body mass index [BMI]) for every bottle of sports drink they drank each day, compared with the weight gain (2 pounds [0.9 kg]) associated with a can of regular soda.[28] According to lead researcher Allison Field of Harvard University, "Sports drinks have an even stronger relationship to weight gain than regular sugary sodas."[28] In other words, relying on sports drinks as the main hydration source when not needed may cause just as much weight gain as regular soda—if not more.

Adding to the confusion, sports drinks provide multiple servings in one bottle, something that is easy to miss. Even the smallest bottles have one and a half servings. Parents may look at the label, read "50 calories," and assume that is the calorie content of the whole bottle. A 32-ounce (948 mL) bottle has a total of 200 calories (four servings); to burn this off, a young athlete would need to run 2 miles (3.2 km) or exercise for a half hour or so on the court with intensity and consistency (time on the bench or waiting between running drills doesn't count).

The Young Athlete as a Target

It may be hard to imagine that your young athletes are targets for sports drink companies, but they are. The heavy promotion of sports drinks to young athletes makes them more interesting and enticing, especially when a professional athlete is doing the endorsing. In 2010, Gatorade was among the *top five* most marketed products to children and teens, while Powerade ranked 26th, according to a 2012 review entitled *Consumption of Sports Drinks by Children and Adolescents.*[29] As soda has declined in popularity, consumption of sports drinks has increased, according to the trade journal *Beverage Digest.*[30] While sports drinks might have a role in a young athlete's exercise program, that role should be limited.

Milk

There's no doubt that milk or a milk alternative like soymilk is needed in an athlete's daily diet. Where else can you get the nutritious combination of protein, calcium, vitamin D, and potassium wrapped into such an economical package? Children and teens who consume three servings of dairy (milk, milk alternative, cheese, yogurt, etc.) each day can meet the lion's share of their nutritional requirements for calcium and vitamin D.[31] Most kids and teens fall short of this goal.

Not only may milk support the growth needs of young athletes; as I discussed in Chapter 2, research has shown that flavored milk can be a good recovery drink after intense exercise.[32] Ten ounces (296 mL) of low-fat chocolate milk will give the young athlete the right combination of protein and carbohydrate, plus extra bone-forming nutrients (about 10 g of protein, 26 g of carbohydrate, 160 calories, 270 mg of calcium, and 125 International Units [IU] of vitamin D). Toss a milk box into that duffel and encourage your athlete to drink it after a long workout. For more on post-exercise nutrition, read Chapter 6.

Juice

Many children and teens love the flavor of juice, and opt for it during the day. According to the AAP, children and teens should limit their juice consumption to 8 to 12 ounces (237 to 355 mL) per day of 100% juice,[33] which offers a source of carbohydrate as well as vitamins. Juice drinks (made with 10% juice or less) are not ideal for exercise, as they offer comparatively little nutrition. And too much juice can sideline an athlete with a stomachache. If your athlete loves juice, consider watering it down.

Soda

Soda contains refined sugar and does not offer the varied sources of carbohydrate for muscles that a sports drink does. It also doesn't offer any nutrients other than sugar. Regular consumption of soda has been associated with weight gain and obesity, and some believe drinking diet soda has the same effect on weight.[34]

Soda and diet soda, such as colas, root beers, cream sodas, and fruit-flavored sodas, may contain caffeine, which is not recommended for children or teens. Caffeine is a stimulant, meaning it accelerates the activity of many organs in the body. It can raise a young athlete's heart rate, blood pressure, speech rate, motor activity, attentiveness, gastric secretions, and temperature, and it may be addictive. It can also disturb sleep and increase anxiety in those with anxiety disorders.[35]

Some sodas also contain phosphoric acid, which is responsible for soda's dark color and acidic taste (though this is masked by sugar or sugar substitutes), which may interfere with bone development and erode tooth enamel. When your young athlete wins that gold medal, you want him or her to stand tall and flash those pearly whites. For all these reasons, soda is not a recommended hydration source for young athletes.

Energy Drinks

Red Bull, Rock Star, Amp, Monster Energy, and 5-Hour Energy are enticing labels for a young and impressionable athlete. Who doesn't want to be a rock star on the field? Why not amp up your speed, agility, and endurance on the court, or be able to sustain enormous amounts of energy and strength? All of this in a bottle sounds too good to be true—and it is.

Energy drinks are one of the fastest-growing segments of drink sales in America, and their popularity is growing among the young.[36] Athletes use energy drinks to rehydrate after a workout, to boost attention and focus during school, to "wake up," or as a beverage at meals. While the promise of endurance, energy, and improved performance contained in an all-in-one drink is tempting, drinking them involves some serious downsides for young athletes.

A high school football coach finally figured out why his varsity lineup wasn't "showing up" on the field. In two separate games, his team tanked in the third quarter, complaining of cramping, headaches, and dehydration. Many of them had to come off the field and sit on the bench. As a result, they lost both games. When he learned that his starters were chugging energy drinks in the locker room prior to game time, he put a stop to it and banned energy drinks.

This is a small example compared to what could go wrong. According to the Substance Abuse and Mental Health Services Administration (SAMHSA), the number of emergency room visits related to energy drink consumption doubled from 2007 to 2011.[37] And up to 50% of teens consume energy drinks, according to a 2011 study published in *Pediatrics*.[38] With the popularity of energy drinks, it's fair to assume the emergency-room numbers will grow.

The problem with energy drinks is linked to the high amounts of caffeine they contain—up to 500 milligrams per bottle. Caffeine can be toxic, even lethal, for kids and teens.[39] In 2007, there were over 5,000 caffeine overdoses in the United States, and 46% of those were in youngsters.[40] Obviously, caffeine toxicity is a big concern for young athletes because in today's world it's easy to go overboard. I stand with the AAP, which says that these high caffeine-containing drinks have *no place* in a child's or adolescent's diet.

What's Brewing Inside?

Is your teen nervous? Overly worried? Can't sit still or settle down? Has trouble sleeping? Has the shakes? Stomach pain? Racing heartbeat? Dehydration? These are signs of too much caffeine, maybe even caffeine intoxication, and it's the body's way of telling your teens that they are drinking too much of it. Silent symptoms such as high blood pressure and increased risk of stroke and heart attack can be brewing inside, unbeknownst to either you or the child.

In a *Consumer Reports* article, 27 of the leading energy drinks that were analyzed had caffeine amounts ranging from 6 to 242 milligrams per serving.[41] Energy drinks may contain more than one serving per container, which can increase the total caffeine intake. Other ingredients such

Table 4-3 Selected Ingredients in Energy Drinks

Ingredient	Proposed Function	Comments
Caffeine	Boosts energy levels; sharpens attention	Effects have not been studied in children or teens; potential negative health effects include increased heart rate, agitation, insomnia, and toxicity; keep intake less than 85 to 100 mg per day (1 cup of strong coffee or 2 regular sodas)
Guarana	Increases energy, enhances physical performance, promotes weight loss	Naturally contains 40–80 mg of caffeine; unknown effect on kids and teens
Sodium	Replaces losses in sweat	Content varies from 25 to 200 mg per cup
Potassium	Replaces losses in sweat	Varies from 30 to 90 mg per cup
Amino acids	Enhances muscle recovery after exercise; *glutamine* enhances immune function; *taurine* makes caffeine more potent; *arginine* causes dilation of the blood vessels	Most children and teens match their protein needs with food; use of amino acids and their effects are not supported in the scientific literature and are discouraged
Various herbals	Claims vary but revolve around better immunity, enhanced athletic performance, and quicker recovery	Check Chapter 7 for specifics; some herbal additives can be lethal

as guarana, a plant extract, naturally contain caffeine (1 g of guarana contains 40 to 80 mg of caffeine), adding to the total amount of caffeine content. Other additives, such as taurine, make caffeine more potent. Others, such as amino acids (protein), vitamins, and electrolytes, claim to enhance athletic performance, but the research to date does not support this. I discuss supplement ingredients in Chapter 7. See Table 4-3 for some of the known contents in energy drinks.

Caffeine intoxication may seem an unlikely problem for your young athletes, but if they are drinking their morning coffee from the local coffee shop, and are having a soda, an afternoon coffee drink, and a shot or two of an energy drink, it's not out of the question—in fact, it's probable. Alicia was heading to the coffee shop before school and ordering a large strong brew, heading back again during her free period for a flavored coffee drink, and downing an energy drink or two before soccer practice, depending on how tired she was. The excessive caffeine intake was giving her insomnia, which created a vicious cycle. She needed more boosts of caffeine during the day to prevent withdrawal symptoms and correct her exhaustion. Alicia was hovering close to toxicity, and she was certainly experiencing side effects. I advised her to substitute a decaffeinated version of her afternoon beverage and nix the energy drinks, as they were most definitely interfering with her sleep and setting the stage for repeat behavior the next day. Eventually, her goal was to wean down to one morning coffee—a better and healthier approach than her current pattern.

Why Aren't Energy Drinks Regulated Like Other Food and Beverages?

Energy drinks are not a food, so they don't fall under traditional regulation by the Food and Drug Administration (FDA). Caffeine is not considered a nutrient, unless it is added to a food (such as soda), in which case it then comes under the jurisdiction of the FDA. Energy drinks are sold under the dietary supplements category, which is regulated by the FDA on a *voluntary* basis. This means energy drink manufacturers and other dietary supplement manufacturers "are not legally required to report 'adverse events' to the FDA, including injuries or illnesses that may be related to the use of their products," according to the Office of the Inspector General at the Department of Health and Human Services, in the executive summary of its Adverse Event Reporting for Dietary Supplements.[42] The FDA monitors safety through voluntary adverse event reporting, reports of labeling claims or misinformation, errant product literature, and only occasional laboratory testing. This fact allows energy drink manufacturers to label caffeine content (or not) and test safety (or not). Currently, scientists, the AAP, and the American Medical Association (AMA) are petitioning for stronger jurisdiction and regulation of energy drinks. For more information, see Chapter 7.

Keeping your young athletes healthy and hydrated means selecting *what* they drink and monitoring *how much* they drink. Be smart and savvy about when to use a sports drink, and keep an eye out for energy drinks and sugary beverages. Above all, pick the drinks that will enhance growth and athletic performance, while minimizing any negative impact on daily living.

Getting Practical with Healthy Drinks

Not every young athlete will do well with drinking water—or a sports drink, for that matter. Nicole was frustrated with her 9-year-old daughter, Anna, a swimmer, who didn't like sports drinks or water very much and was forgetting to drink at practice. Nicole was sure Anna was getting dehydrated and needed some ideas to improve the situation. Anna liked 100% orange juice, so Nicole diluted it with water, and even tried mixing it with sparkling water. Nicole also tried experimenting with homemade sports drinks (see below), using orange juice as a base.

I suggested that Nicole give Anna some drinking guidelines: her labeled bottle needed to perch at the edge of the pool or at the end of the lane where she was swimming so the drink would be calling her name at breaks. Anna was to take two to four gulps of fluid at a time. Nicole also asked the coach to help remind Anna to drink. With all these measures in place, Anna got into the routine of drinking on her own, and it became a nonissue.

Do-It-Yourself Sports Drinks

Some families enjoy making homemade versions of sports drinks, which gives them the flexibility with ingredients and enables them to avoid artificial sweeteners, colors, and unknown chemicals while also saving money. Try the following recipes. You can change the juice component to the flavor preferences of your young athlete.

Lemonade Sports Drink

¼ cup (60 mL) lemonade plus 2 tablespoons (30 mL) of lemon juice

¼ cup (48 g) sugar

¼ teaspoon (1 mL) salt

¼ cup (60 mL) hot water

3½ cups (830 mL) cold water

In a pitcher or quart-size water jug, add the sugar and salt to the hot water; stir until sugar and salt are dissolved. Add the lemonade, lemon juice, and cold water. Mix well. Makes 1 quart (.96 L).

Strawberry Lime Sports Drink

4 to 6 whole strawberries, cleaned, hulled, and muddled (smashed)

¼ cup (60 mL) limeade plus 2 tablespoons (30 mL) of lime juice

¼ cup (48 g) sugar

¼ teaspoon (1 mL) salt

¼ cup (60 mL) hot water

3½ cups (830 mL) cold water

In a pitcher or quart-size water jug, add the sugar and salt to the hot water; shake or stir until sugar and salt are dissolved. Add the strawberries, limeade, lime juice, and cold water. Mix well. Makes 1 quart (.96 L).

Watermelon Slushy

6 or 7 cups (or more) seedless watermelon, roughly chopped

24 ounces (711 mL) plain seltzer water

¼ cup (48 g) sugar

¼ teaspoon (1 mL) salt

In a blender, add the watermelon, seltzer, sugar, and salt. Blend well. Makes about 1 quart (.96 L). *Note:* Add more seltzer for a thinner beverage.

Hot Tip!

Pour your homemade sports drinks into popsicle molds. Athletes performing workouts in hot and humid weather deserve a frozen treat, and these treats will count toward recovery hydration.

Keep in mind that many foods have high water content and can be useful in helping kids and teens stay hydrated. Juicy fruits like watermelon, applesauce, ripe peaches, citrus fruits, strawberries, star fruit, and melon are over 90% water. Think about vegetables, too. Good choices are cucumber, iceberg lettuce, celery, radish, tomatoes, green pepper, spinach, baby carrots, and cauliflower, which also weigh in at about 90% water. Yogurt and milk are 80% water, and soups and vegetable juice have high water and sodium content as well.

While hydration may look simple, statistics tell us that many kids and teens are falling behind on fluids and making the wrong beverage choices. Becoming dehydrated is something all young athletes want to avoid. Not only does it make them feel unwell, it hinders their athletic performance and can be dangerous to their health. Help your athlete by outlining a personalized drinking plan and set guidelines for appropriate drink types. And make sure your athlete checks his hydration status regularly to stay in tip-top form.

Notes

1. Sexton M. "Beat the heat: athletic training prof offers hydration tips." University of South Carolina. http://www.sc.edu/news/newsarticle.php?nid =4313#.U3vCCq1dWuZ.
2. Manz F, Wentz A, and Sichert-Hellert W. "The most essential nutrient: defining the adequate intake of water." *J Pediatr.* 141 (2002): 587–592.
3. Holliday MA and Segar WE. "The maintenance need for water in parenteral fluid therapy." *Pediatrics.* 19 (1957): 823–832.
4. Institute of Medicine. *DRI, dietary reference intakes for water, potassium, sodium, chloride, and sulfate.* Washington, DC: National Academies Press, 2005.
5. Rowland T. "Fluid replacement requirements for child athletes." *Sports Med.* 41 (2011): 279–288.
6. Rowland T. "Thermoregulation during exercise in the heat in children: old concepts revisited." *J Appl Physiol.* 105 (2008): 718–724.
7. Bergeron MF, McLeod KS, and Coyle JF. "Core body temperature during competition in the heat: National Boys' 14s Junior Tennis Championships." *Br J Sports Med.* 41 (2007): 779–783.
8. Gilchrist J. "Heat illness among high school athletes—United States, 2005–2009." Centers for Disease Control. *MMWR.* 59 (2010): 1009–1013.

9. Mayo Clinic. *Heatstroke: First Aid.* http://www.mayoclinic.org/first-aid/first-aid-heatstroke/basics/art-20056655.

10. Falk B and Dolan R. "Temperature regulation and elite young athletes." *Med Sport Sci.* 56 (2011): 126–149.

11. Wilk B, Yuzio H, and Bar-Or O. "Effect of body hypohydration on aerobic performance of boys who exercise in the heat." *Med Sci Sports Exerc.* 34 (2002): S48.

12. Rowland T. "Fluid replacement requirements for child athletes," op. cit, p. 285.

13. Ibid.

14. Barclay L. "AAP Update on guidelines for heat safety in exercising youth." *Medscape.* www.medscape.org/viewarticle/748003.

15. Rowland T. "Fluid replacement requirements for child athletes," op. cit, p. 282.

16. Arnaoutis G, Kavouras SA, Kotsis YP, Tsekouras YE, Makrillos M, and Bardis CN. "Ad libitum fluid intake does not prevent dehydration in suboptimally hydrated young soccer players during a training session of a summer camp." *Int J Sport Nutr Exerc Metab.* 23 (2013): 245–251.

17. Wilk B, Timmons BW, and Bar-Or O. "Voluntary fluid intake, hydration status, and aerobic performance of adolescent athletes in the heat." *Appl Physiol Nutr Metab.* 35 (2010): 834–841.

18. American College of Sports Medicine, Sawka MN, Burke LM, Eichner ER, Maughan RJ, Montain SJ, and Stachenfeld NS. "American College of Sports Medicine position stand. Exercise and fluid replacement." *Med Sci Sports Exerc.* 39 (2007): 377–390.

19. Yeargin SW, Casa DJ, Judelson DA, McDermott BP, Ganio MS, Lee EC, Lopez RM, Stearns RL, Anderson JM, Armstrong LE, Kraemer WJ, and Maresh CM. "Thermoregulatory responses and hydration practices in heat-acclimatized adolescents during preseason high school football." *J Athl Train.* 45 (2010): 136–146.

20. Armstrong LE. "Hydration assessment techniques." *Nutr Rev.* 63 (2005): S40–S54.

21. U.S. Department of Agriculture and U.S. Department of Health and Human Services. "*Dietary Guidelines for Americans, 2015.*" Available at: http://www.health.gov/dietaryguidelines/2015-scientific-report/PDFs/Scientific-Report-of-the-2015-Dietary-Guidelines-Advisory-Committee.pdf

22. Birch LL. "Development of food preferences." *Annu Rev Nutr.* 19 (1999): 41–62.

23. Rowland T. "Fluid replacement requirements for child athletes," op. cit, p. 284.

24. Latif R. "Premium hydration overtakes enhanced water." *BevNet.* http://www.bevnet.com/magazine/issue/2013/premium-hydration-overtakes-enhanced-water.
25. Committee on Nutrition and the Council on Sports Medicine and Fitness, American Academy of Pediatrics. "Sports drinks and energy drinks for children and adolescents: are they appropriate?" *Pediatrics.* 127 (2011): 1182–1189.
26. Herold L. "Are sports drinks fueling our young athletes or fueling the national obesity epidemic?" University of Minnesota News: Driven to Discover. http://www1.umn.edu/news/expert-alerts/2012/UR_CONTENT_406179.html.
27. Harris JL, Schwartz MB, and Brownell KD. *Sugary Drink FACTS. Evaluating Sugary Drink Nutrition and Marketing to Youth.* Hartford, CT: Yale Rudd Center for Food Policy and Obesity, 2011.
28. Zimmerman R. "Sports drinks, not just sodas, drive up weight in teens." Medscape. http://www.medscape.com/viewarticle/791326.
29. Story M, Klein L, and Robert Wood Johnson Foundation. "Consumption of sports drinks by children and adolescents. A research review." Robert Wood Johnson Foundation. http://www.rwjf.org/en/research-publications/find-rwjf-research/2012/06/consumption-of-sports-drinks-by-children-and-adolescents.html.
30. Blanc M. "US soda sales: should Coca-Cola and PepsiCo be worried?" BidnessEtc. http://www.bidnessetc.com/21356-coca-cola-ko-pepsico-pep-news-us-soda-sales-decline/.
31. U.S. Department of Agriculture and U.S. Department of Health and Human Services, op. cit., p. 51.
32. Pritchett K and Pritchett R. "Chocolate milk: a post-exercise recovery beverage for endurance sports." *Med Sport Sci.* 59 (2012): 127–134.
33. American Academy of Pediatrics. "Fruit juice and your child's diet." healthychildren.org. http://www.healthychildren.org/English/healthy-living/nutrition/Pages/Fruit-Juice-and-Your-Childs-Diet.aspx.
34. Swithers SE. "Artificial sweeteners produce the counterintuitive effect of inducing metabolic derangements." *Trends Endocrinol Metab.* 24 (2013): 431–441.
35. Seifert SM, Schaechter JL, Hershorin ER, and Lipschultz SE. "Health effects of energy drinks on children, adolescents, and young adults." *Pediatrics,* 127 (2011): 511–528.
36. Blanc, op. cit.
37. Substance Abuse and Mental Health Services Association. "1 in 10 energy drink-related emergency department visits results in hospitalization." *DAWN*

Report. http://www.samhsa.gov/data/spotlight/spot124-energy-drinks-2014 .pdf.

38. Seifert, op. cit, p. 515.
39. Ibid.
40. Substance Abuse and Mental Health Services Association, op. cit.
41. Consumer Reports. "The buzz on energy-drink caffeine." ConsumerReports .org. http://www.consumerreports.org/cro/magazine/2012/12/the-buzz-on -energy-drink-caffeine/index.htm.
42. U.S. Health and Human Services, Office of the Inspector General, 2001. "Adverse event reporting for dietary supplements. An inadequate safety valve." http://oig.hhs.gov/oei/reports/oei-01-00-00180.pdf.

PART II

Play-by-Play Eating

CHAPTER 5

Game Plan—One, Two, Three Meals!

If you fail to prepare, you're prepared to fail.
—Mark Spitz, Olympic gold medalist in swimming

Debbie knew she had to have a meal at the ready when her 18-year-old daughter, Lauren, a club volleyball player, came home from practice. After a 2-hour practice and a 45-minute drive home, Lauren arrived at a late dinner hour and was generally tired, cranky, and hungry. If Debbie didn't have dinner ready, her daughter would be in the pantry and refrigerator, hunting for food. Yet getting a meal on the table wasn't easy. "I have three other kids who also have sports and other after-school activities, so I have to have a plan—and every day may be different, depending on what's going on," explained Debbie.

According to a publication from the National Center on Addiction and Substance Abuse called *The Importance of Family Dinner VIII*, only six out of 10 families sit together for the evening meal, and this number takes a nose dive when there are teenagers in the house.[1] According to a study from the *American Journal of Lifestyle Medicine*, one third of teens skip breakfast.[2] What this research tells us is that making meals, eating together, and instilling the importance of regular meals is no easy task for American families. In fact, it's a huge challenge.

While some parents are lost in the kitchen, lacking the skills to plan and cook meals, others are strapped for time and instead head to the drive-through window on the way home from practice or stock the pantry with convenience items. Juggling the demands of cooking, the time limitations, and the need for high-quality meals can place added stress on even the most organized and well-intentioned parent.

And yet the underlying issue remains: nutritious meals are the backbone of athletic training and performance.

This chapter will help you develop or revamp your game plan when it comes to preparing meals. I will cover the science behind meals and their benefits; showcase overall nutrition, portions, and food group balance; and show you how to make your kitchen skills (whatever they may be) work for you and your athlete. Then I'll review your options for getting healthy meals on the table fast. Since eating food prepared outside the home is a reality for the families of busy athletes, I'll cover healthy versions of takeout and fast food, as well as tips for dining out. My intention is to make healthy meals easy and stress-free for everyone.

Focus on the Family Meal

"I'm not sure which is harder—planning meals ahead of time, cooking them, or getting everyone together at once," said Karen, a mom of three active kids. "It just seems that my dinner hour is pure chaos." Karen isn't alone. For many parents and their athletes, dinner represents the culmination of a long, tiring day when family members are stressed, impatient, and hungry. And Karen was falling behind in her efforts to get good, nutritious meals on the table. She didn't have a master plan for her weekly meals, and she often ran out of time to cook. While she scrambled in the kitchen, her hungry athletes complained, foraged in the pantry for something to eat, or both. Karen needed a game plan.

Why should parents like Karen break their backs to make family meals? There's a very good reason: research tells us that arranging for the family to have meals together may help facilitate raising emotionally and physically healthy children. Regular family meals—kids and teens sitting together with one or both parents, three or more times per week—have been linked with children's improved health, academic success, healthier eating and body weight, and improved self-esteem.[3]

Family meals may help reduce risk-taking behaviors in teens, such as drinking, driving, and disordered eating. This may be particularly important for the teen athlete; a 2012 review study published in the *Journal of Sports Science and Medicine* found that teen athletes had higher rates of alcohol use than nonathletes.[4] A nutritious meal and a positive meal environment—one that is pleasant, engaging, and supportive—can go a long way toward helping your athlete stay on course with nutrition, development, and healthy lifestyle behaviors.

Making Everyday Food Good Food

Family meals are invaluable for your athlete, but what about the food? How can you take what you've learned earlier in this book and apply it to everyday meals? A few nutrition basics, such as balancing the food groups and serving reasonable portion sizes, will help you plan and cook tasty meals that support good health.

Balancing the Food Groups

There are five different food groups outlined by the United States Department of Agriculture (USDA) that identify the types of food to include in your daily meals.[5] You can view them at ChooseMyPlate.gov. I've added two additional food categories—oils and desserts—for you to keep track of and manage. These will help facilitate healthy eating for your family. The goal is to have a reasonable plan for getting each of the following food groups into your children's meals and snacks each day.

Lean Protein. Foods with lean protein include meat, poultry, seafood, beans, nuts, seeds, and eggs. These foods come from animals and plants, and contain an excellent source of protein. Some foods from animal sources, such as bacon, sausage, or ribs, are naturally higher in fat (and thus high in calories) than others like skinless chicken breast or fish. *Choose lean sources of protein* most of the time. Seafood contains monounsaturated fats, so try to plan for 6 to 8 ounces (170 to 227 g) of fish per week. Processed meats include added sodium, so keep an eye on the amounts you serve if you're concerned about sodium intake. Many of the foods in this group are also good sources of iron, zinc, and vitamin B$_{12}$.

Dairy. Sources of dairy include milk, yogurt, cheeses, and nondairy substitutes such as soymilk. Dairy foods, which are good sources of protein and carbohydrate, contain varying levels of fat. For example, whole milk contains more fat than low-fat or skim milk. *Stick to lower fat dairy products.* Because dairy foods contain both carbs and protein, they are an ideal recovery food after intense physical activity. Foods in this group also provide a good source of calcium and if fortified, a good source of vitamin D.

Fruit. Fruit can be fresh, frozen, canned, or dried, or in the form of 100% fruit juice. Limit juice amounts to 8 to 12 ounces (237 to 355 mL) per day. There are loads of fiber in whole fruit, as well as potassium, folic acid, and vitamin C. When planning and serving meals, *fill half the plate with fruits and vegetables.*

Vegetables. Vegetables can be fresh, frozen, canned, or dehydrated, or in the form of 100% vegetable juice. They provide a wide variety of nutrients, so vegetables are further categorized into five subgroups: dark green vegetables (broccoli and kale); starchy (corn and potatoes); red and orange (tomatoes and carrots); beans and peas (kidney beans and split peas); and other vegetables (artichokes and Brussels sprouts). The starchy vegetables and beans and peas subgroups offer the athlete an excellent source of complex carbohydrates. Vegetables also provide key nutrients such as fiber, vitamins A and C, folic acid, and potassium. It's worth repeating the above suggestion: *fill half the plate with fruits and vegetables.*

Grains. Cereals, breads, pasta, and rice are divided into two types: whole grains and refined grains. *Whole grains* contain the intact grain kernel, including the bran, germ, and endosperm. These are the most desirable grains for health, appetite control, and prevention of chronic disease. *Eat half of your daily grains from a whole-grain source,* such as brown rice, whole wheat bread, and oatmeal. *Refined grains* have been milled, removing the bran and germ. This process also removes fiber, B vitamins, and iron. Manufacturers add B vitamins and iron back to the product after processing, in a process called *enrichment*; this isn't usually the case for fiber, although more manufacturers are highlighting this important nutrient in their refined products. Make sure refined grains are enriched, an especially important consideration for gluten-free products, which may not be.

Oils. Oils provide the diet with important nutrients, such as fat-soluble vitamins and the healthy omega-3 fatty acids. Hard fats such as butter are solid at room temperature and contain saturated fats. Regardless of the source, fats provide considerable calories. While you'll want to *eat more oils than solid fats*, you'll also want to keep a cap on the amounts.

Desserts. It is important that you understand how to balance desserts. Whether you offer your children a dessert routinely is up to you, but many families do better with some sort of policy about desserts. Over the course of a week, you can *offer your athlete an average of one or possibly even two desserts a day* if he or she is very active and has high calorie needs. There may be no dessert on some days and more than one on others. The goal is to make dessert a small part of the overall diet. If your athlete eats a lot of sweets, it's a good idea to cut back on some of them, as they will crowd out the nutrient-rich foods he or she needs. Always keep your eye on the long-term impact of desserts. Those huge bowls of ice cream at the end of the day can turn into a habitual indulgence.

It's a Balancing Act

Thoughtful meal planning should target *at least four* of the five food groups (protein, dairy, fruit, vegetable, and grain) in every meal—breakfast, lunch, and dinner. If you can include all five in all three meals, terrific! This strategy alone will increase the likelihood that your athletes will get the important nutrients they need every day. When I plan meals, I always start with the protein source and work from there. I then plan the vegetable and/or fruit, grain, and dairy. Weekends tend to be our planned dessert nights (often it's ice cream), and I stock my kitchen with healthy fats (olive oil, safflower oil, and canola oil).

When you use a food group approach to meal planning, it's really a matter of filling in the blanks. For example, breakfast may include scrambled eggs, whole wheat toast, strawberries, and a glass of low-fat milk. Lunch may be a deli meat sandwich (containing grain, protein, dairy, vegetables, and fat) with a side of carrots and yogurt. Dinner could be chicken, green beans, banana slices, quinoa, and milk. The old saying, "Variety is the spice of life," holds true with food. Keep the variety coming within the different food groups, as it will keep your athletes more interested in eating and help you successfully cover their nutrition needs.

Practical Tips for Balanced Meals

- Include fruit and milk (or a milk substitute) with every meal, even dinner. It's a great way to round out the meal, and many athletes will readily eat these foods.
- Thumbs down on veggies? If your athlete isn't a fan, continue to offer them anyway. It may simply be a matter of time before he or she warms up to certain veggies. In the meantime, add fruits to your menu—they are a decent stand-in for veggies and contain similar nutrients.
- Start your planning for each meal with a protein source, whether it's meat, fish, beans, or eggs. This focus will help you meet your family's protein needs, avoid erratic protein intake, and space protein consumption evenly throughout the day.
- Combination foods like lasagna, pizza, and other casseroles cover more than one food group and count toward the overall food group balance. Just add a side of milk, vegetable, and/or fruit to these entrees.
- If your athlete loves bread and other refined grains, gradually work in whole grains. For instance, mix white and brown rice, or whole-wheat and regular pasta, in a 1:1 ratio; purchase whole white wheat bread (made from a wheat that is white in color rather than brown, which is milder in flavor, and contains the nutritional profile of traditional whole wheat). For dessert, try baking cookies and brownies with whole-wheat flour.
- Stock your pantry and refrigerator with healthy fats, such as olive oil, safflower, or canola oil. Use them for cooking, baking, and salad dressings. Butter, shortening, and stick margarine are high in saturated fats, so a little goes a long way.

- Food repeats are boring. Don't offer the same foods over and over, like bananas and green beans. Challenge yourself to increase the variety within each food group.

Breakfast

Start your athlete's day with a protein-packed, carb-rich breakfast. You've heard it before: "Breakfast is the most important meal of the day." Why? Breakfast breaks the overnight fasting period and sucks up all the stomach acids that accumulate overnight, "jump starts" your athlete's calorie-burning engine (metabolism), and kicks the appetite hormones into gear so that they can alert your athlete when to eat. Unfortunately, not all athletes are interested in eating early in the morning, but we know that breakfast provides many benefits for health, wellness, body weight, academic success, and more.

For athletes who have sports practice in the morning before school or for some other reason have little time to eat, provide a few grab-and-go options that they can eat on the fly or in the classroom. Here are some of my go-to breakfast combos—they are packed with protein, carbs, and nutrients:

- Gorp (dry cereal, nuts, dried fruit, and/or chocolate bits) packed in small baggies
- 6 ounces (177 mL) of Greek yogurt and a banana
- Single-serve cup of peanut butter and a large sliced apple
- A packaged cheese stick and a high-protein granola bar, such as a KIND bar
- Overnight oatmeal (mix ½ cup [64 g] of oats, 1 cup [237 mL] of milk, 2 tablespoons [30 g] of dried fruit, and 1 tablespoon [15 g] of chia seeds in a container and refrigerate, covered, overnight; warm it up and top with 1 to 2 tablespoons [15 to 30 g] of nuts in the morning).
- Muffin and two clementines (or one other piece of medium-sized fruit)
- Two mini-bagels with nut butter and a milk box

- A peanut-butter-and-jam sandwich on whole-wheat bread
- Two hard-boiled eggs and 1 cup (237 mL) of 100% juice

In a pinch, a liquid meal can be a nutritious alternative. Look for balanced instant breakfast-type beverages or make your own blended smoothie drink using milk, yogurt, frozen fruit, fresh spinach or kale, and/or 100% juice.

Lunch

If your athletes have games after school, what they eat at lunch will be critical. Greasy pizza is not a good choice on game day. You can either pack their lunches yourself or have them purchase lunch at school. Since brown-bag lunches can be just as unhealthy as the cafeteria's chicken nuggets and French fries, and lunch is fuel for the game, I asked Katie Sullivan Morford, a registered dietitian and author of *Best Lunch Box Ever*, to share her suggestions.[6] Parents can step up the "nutritious" angle in the lunch box every day with these six steps:

1. Start with the main course: sandwich, salad, or an insulated container filled with dinner leftovers (all protein-heavy, of course).
2. Add a fruit: whole, seasonal options preferred. Make fruit easy to grab and eat by cutting and peeling it before packing.
3. Add a vegetable: sides of raw veggies or salad are more enticing with a dip or dressing, so pack a small container for these. If your main course contains veggies, this step is optional.
4. Include a satisfying side or snack: avoid the usual crunchy snacks. Try exotic nuts, homemade popcorn, or dried fruit—you'll raise the nutritional value and skip the "processed" factor.
5. Don't forget a drink: water or milk preferred.
6. Surprise your athlete with an occasional sweet or loving touch: including a homemade goodie (chocolate chip cookie or brownie) or even just writing a funny note or joke can make lunch a positive part of the day.

Alternatively, if your athletes will purchase lunch at school, take a quick glance at the menu and offer some suggestions that will prep them for the competition, keeping in mind the need for carbohydrates and protein and limited fat. A lean meat sandwich on whole-grain bread and/or a bean-based soup, a piece of fruit, and a glass of low-fat milk are good options. If they prefer a hot meal, suggest the chicken breast, baked potato, green beans, and fruit cup, with low-fat milk or yogurt on the side, or something similar. Advise them to steer clear of desserts, ice cream, fried food, and bags of chips on game day.

The Pre-Competition Meal

The pre-competition meal (one that occurs 3 to 4 hours before the competition) should provide less fat and fiber in order to avoid fullness and discomfort. Instead, it should provide lean protein sources and low-fat dairy options, and should avoid fried foods like fried chicken, French fries, and chips. Your athletes shouldn't eat loads of fiber at this meal, either. Most importantly, they should eat foods that they know their bodies tolerate before a game.

What about the night before a competition? There will be plenty of time to digest this food, so the focus should be on a well-rounded, nutritious meal. Good options are a pasta meal, such as spaghetti with marinara sauce or a deep-dish pizza with a side of salad, or a Mexican meal such as fajitas with veggies plus a side of rice and beans. Remember, children and young teen athletes don't "load" glycogen in their muscles like adults do, as discussed in Chapter 2, so the carb-loading approach isn't necessary. The best bet is to provide a tasty meal representing a balance of food groups to fuel your athlete sufficiently for tomorrow's demands.

Serving Sizes

In our world of portion distortion and "bigger is better," many athletes are overeating. It is not hard to do this, as the sizes of many food offerings have increased substantially over the past three decades. The old bagel was the size of a tuna fish can; the new bagel is almost three times bigger. A standard soda was 12 ounces (355 mL); now you see twice that size in vending machines—and up to 32 ounces (almost 1 L) in convenience stores. Even the useful sports drink has exploded in size. Your athlete needs to understand what normal serving sizes of food and drink look like.

Table 5-1 Food Group Serving Sizes and Minimum Daily Intake

Group	Serving Size	Daily Amount Based on Child's Age	Comments
Protein	3 ounces	8 years: 4 oz 9–13 years: 5 oz 14–18 years: 5 oz (female) 14–18 years: 6.5 oz (male)	One-ounce equivalents are: 1 ounce meat, poultry or fish; ¼ cup cooked beans; 1 tablespoon nut butter; ½ ounce nuts or seeds; 1 egg
Dairy	1 cup	8 years: 2.5 cups 9–18 years: 3 cups	1 cup milk or yogurt; 1½ ounces cheese; ⅓ cup shredded cheese; 2 ounces processed cheese; 1 cup pudding
Grains	½ cup	8 years: 2.5 oz 9–13 years (female): 5 oz 9–13 years (male): 6 oz 14–18 years (female): 6 oz 14–18 years (male): 8 oz	1 slice (1 oz) bread; ½ cup cooked pasta, rice, cereal or other grain; 1 cup (weight varies) ready-to-eat cereal
Fruit	1 cup	8 years: 1–1.5 cups 9–13 years: 1.5 cups 14–18 years (female): 1.5 cups 14–18 years (male): 2 cups	1 cup fresh, frozen, canned or 100% juice; ½ cup dried fruit
Vegetables	1 cup	8 years: 1.5 cups 9–13 years (female): 2 cups 9–13 years (male): 2.5 cups 14–18 years (female): 2.5 cups 14–18 years (male): 3 cups	1 cup fresh, frozen, canned vegetables or vegetable juice; 2 cups raw leafy greens
Fats	1 teaspoon	8 years: 4 teaspoons 9–13 years: 5 teaspoons 14–18 years (female): 5 teaspoons 14–18 years (male): 6 teaspoons	1 tablespoon of vegetable oil equals 3 teaspoons 1 ounce of nuts equals ~3 teaspoons 2 tablespoons of peanut butter equals 4 teaspoons 1 tablespoon of margarine equals 2.5 teaspoons

Source: Adapted from: http://www.choosemyplate.gov/food-groups/.

Table 5-1 offers standard serving sizes for each food group, along with the amount needed each day to meet the minimum nutrient requirements and their various food options.

Reading Food Labels. One way to understand healthy portions is to know how to read the Nutrition Facts label provided on food product packaging. Understanding and using this label will help you make thoughtful food choices. The serving size information at the top of the label sets the basis for the calories and nutrients detailed on the rest of the label. The number of calories and amounts of other major nutrients such as protein, fat, carbohydrate, fiber, cholesterol, sodium, and sugar, based on one serving, are also listed. Many products, such as sports drinks, contain more than one serving. One serving of a sports drink is 8 ounces (237 mL), but many bottles contain 24 ounces (710 mL), or three servings, so you need to multiply the value of the nutrients by a factor of 3 to get the total number of calories and the amounts of other nutrients that the bottle contains. The Daily Value (DV) expresses the amount of nutrient content per serving compared to the daily requirements: a DV of 20% or more is a high source of a particular nutrient, while less than 5% is a low source. Reading the Nutrition Facts label helps you identify portions and calories, meet the mark on nutrients, and even trim ones that we should eat in limited amounts, like fat and sugar.

The Mealtime Environment: Keeping It Happy

Providing your athlete with the right nutrition is critical, but the context in which food is served is just as important. Often the stresses involved in getting a meal on the table can turn a happy family gathering into a dreaded obligation. Not only do you need to keep health a priority at the table; it's also important to keep the vibe pleasant. Kids and teens who are pressured to eat more food, who are reprimanded for eating too much or making poor choices, or who have to endure fighting or other adversity at the table will not walk away feeling good about the experience. You want your young athletes to look forward to family meals and walk away associating a nutritious meal with happiness and stability, so that they reap the social-emotional benefits I mentioned earlier.

Your Feeding Style

I'm a big believer in the *authoritative* feeding style, in which the parent takes on the job of determining meals and menus, sets up the timing and location of eating, and lets the child make reasonable food choices from what is offered. I cover this concept in great detail in my first book, *Fearless Feeding: How to Raise Healthy Eaters from High Chair to High School.*[7]

Many parents use other feeding styles, some of which may get in the way of healthy eating. The *authoritarian* parent (not to be confused with the *authoritative* parent) may determine portions and make up the athletes' plate for them, tell them to eat more, stop them from having seconds, excessively control sweets or junk food, and give little credence to hunger, fullness, or food preferences. Such parents may actually create resistance to healthy eating, or their athletes may develop unhealthy eating patterns and gain or drop weight.

Permissive parents, in contrast, go in the opposite direction, saying yes to everything or being loose with timing and boundaries around food. As a result, sweets and junk food eating may be out of control, and good nutrition habits a nagging ideal rather than a reality. Because permissive parents allow kids to eat almost anything, unhealthy eating habits may develop, and the athlete may incur weight issues.

All in all, your goal should be a feeding style that helps you raise an athlete who knows how to eat, what to eat, and when to eat. The authoritative style gets you to that place faster. Much of the advice in this book for feeding your athlete reflects this authoritative approach.

Timing of Meals

Young athletes should eat meals every 5 or 6 hours, with snacks spaced in between—for example, breakfast at 7:00 a.m., lunch at 12:30 p.m., and dinner at 6:00 p.m., with snacks at 10:00 a.m. and 3:00 p.m. Of course, snacks will vary, based on your athlete's age (children need two or three snacks per day, and teens need one or two, based on activity), something I'll discuss in detail in the next chapter. This feeding structure will help your athlete in two ways: it will offer an array of nutrients spaced evenly throughout the day, and it will curtail excessive hunger. Ideally, meals should take place at a routine place—a table or island counter where the family can gather. Sitting in front of the TV or eating in the car or alone in a bedroom does not deliver the positive benefits of eating together as a family.

Cooking When Time Is Tight

Whether or not you consider yourself adept in the kitchen, the daily grind of getting meals on the table can be stressful. In a survey of adult cooking skills, 28% of people said they didn't know how to cook, citing lack of knowledge and time.[8] Another survey found that 42% of parents spent time teaching their children how to cook.[9] While this number is encouraging, the reality is that a fair number of parents can't cook, and because of this, they don't teach their kids to cook.

If you're in the "can't cook" camp, meals will be harder, but certainly not impossible. There are many ways to approach cooking a meal, from traditional "from scratch" meals to meals that use healthy prepared items. This section is all about speedy, nutritious meals that keep stress at arm's length, and are good for both you and your athlete.

Mostly Homemade

Cooking from scratch offers the ultimate control of ingredients and nutrition. Every ingredient, from protein and fiber to sugar and fat, can be enhanced or emphasized, or modified, cut down, or eliminated. Many families and school lunch programs are opting to make food from scratch. Many people agree that homemade tastes better.

But preparing homemade food takes time. One way to make the most of your time is to double- or triple-size your recipes. For example, if you make a killer spaghetti sauce, double the batch and freeze it in freezer bags. You can do the same with lasagna, chili, breads, soups, and more. For subsequent meals, you'll need just a quick reheat on the stove or in the oven.

"I try to keep meals as simple as possible," says Garrett Weber-Gayle, two-time Olympic gold medalist in swimming. "My wife and I make two types of beans and two or three types of grains like brown rice or barley at the beginning of the week, and use them in meals throughout the week," he said. "We like to make a big salad and pile on the beans and grains."

You can also repurpose your food to streamline meals and reduce time. A whole chicken for one meal can be retooled into sandwiches, chicken salad, or chicken soup for another meal or two.

Semi-Homemade

Take shortcuts by using prepared foods such as precooked chicken strips, rice, jarred spaghetti sauce, fresh bakery dough, enchilada sauce, and bagged salad greens. Prepared items can speed up meal prep while keeping meals nutritious. Some of my favorites include meat lasagna using jarred spaghetti sauce and no-cook lasagna noodles, precooked chicken strips on top of a Caesar salad or in burritos, and premade dough from the grocer for a semi-homemade pizza or calzone. One of my fastest semi-homemade meals is a stir-fry using frozen raw shrimp, pre-cut veggies from the supermarket, and Japanese soba noodles—it's ready in less than 30 minutes.

Prepared (with an Eye on Health)

Another way to prepare meals fast is to opt for foods from the grocer or freezer that need just a quick warm-up. For example, pick up a roasted chicken and add frozen veggies and instant brown rice. Or try a soup from the deli and whip up a grilled ham and cheese sandwich. Many other "healthy" foods can be found in the freezer section, including ready-to-go stir-fry entrees, hamburger patties or turkey meatballs, and precooked frozen entrees. If you're buying an entrée, try to find one that offers a lot of vegetables, or add a side salad or piece of fruit. Many healthier frozen entrees focus on lower calories and may not provide enough for the athlete, so add a glass of milk, a salad, and/or some fruit to round out the meal.

Make Ahead

The "make ahead" cooking approach helps you get the main meal started so it cooks itself, especially when you can't be at home. The slow cooker can be useful on some of your busiest nights; you can slow cook food throughout the day and have it ready in the evening. Some of my favorite items to slow cook are inexpensive cuts of beef, dried pinto or black beans, and chicken thighs or breasts. The slow cooker has made a comeback in recent years, and there are many terrific resources available. Three of my favorite resources are Cooking Light's *105 Favorite Slow Cooker Favorites* found on the *Cooking Light* website, Betty Crocker's *Slow Cooker Cookbook*, and One Pot: 120+ Easy Meals from Your Skillet, Slow Cooker, Stockpot, and More by Editors of Martha Stewart Living. These three will definitely help you get beyond pot roast.

Another make-ahead approach is to batch-cook and freeze meal items—lasagna or enchiladas, or soups, stews, and chili. Double or triple your recipe and cook it up. After you serve a single batch for dinner, package, label, and stick the extra entrée(s) in the freezer for another day. You can even combine homemade and semi-homemade cooking with this fast, reheatable option. I have used this strategy to make enchiladas, lasagna, and beef stew. It requires a little bit of planning to calculate and purchase the extra ingredients, but it's worth it when you can pull out a homemade frozen entrée and have it reheating in the oven while you taxi your athlete home.

Keep It Simple

Sometimes simple is the best tactic. Breakfast for dinner (known as "brinner" in my house) or soup and a sandwich can be a perfectly acceptable solution to a busy night of sporting events. Every now and then, I announce a YOYO ("You're on your own") night, letting family members pull a meal together themselves, making sure they include the important food groups. A cheese quesadilla with fruit and raw veggies or a pre-bagged salad shaken out on top of blue corn chips and topped with beans, cheese, and salsa can be a quick and satisfying meal. Sometimes it's a Must-Go night (a silly name for leftovers—they must go!) to clean out the fridge. Just make sure your athlete embellishes with fruit, veggies, and a dairy or nondairy substitute.

Getting Meals on the Table

Now you understand the myriad ways to approach cooking for your athlete, the best foods to prepare, and the balance to strike for meals. You also know how to keep the mealtime environment positive. These are the ingredients for successful meals night after night and day after day. Now it's time to make them happen.

Warning: if you're running to the grocery store more than once or twice a week, it's safe to say you don't have a good meal planning system in place. Running back and forth to the grocery store cuts into one of your most precious resources: time. To streamline your meal planning, you need to have a sense of the rhythm and flow in your week, as this will drive your cooking approach and meal content.

I helped Julie, a busy mom of three, with her mealtime game plan, keeping in mind the demands of her career and the needs of two active high school athletes. We mapped out her week, streamlining her driving and work demands and sporting event obligations. Here's what we came up with:

Day of Week	Activities	Dinner Timing	Type of Meal/Ideas
Monday	Work day Sport practice; driving	6:30 p.m.	Freeze-ahead: enchiladas with fruit and milk
Tuesday	No work After-school Game	5:30 p.m.	Semi-homemade: grilled chicken, couscous, bagged salad, strawberries, milk
Wednesday	Work day Late practice; driving	7:45 p.m.	Make ahead: slow-cooked beans with tortillas, cheese and Mexican toppings
Thursday	No work Carpool; no driving	6:00 p.m.	Make ahead: batch cook three homemade lasagnas and freeze two for later
Friday	Work half-day Game	Flexible	Super simple: YOYO, or kids eat with friends

"Getting a handle on my schedule each week has really helped relieve my stress," says Julie. "When I get away from planning ahead, the stress goes up and our meals suffer."

Breakfast and lunch involve a rotation of staple items—breakfast cereals, eggs, bread, lunchmeat, fruit, dairy products. But dinner is a different story. Many parents (myself included) find dinner to be more difficult, as it involves the biggest variables. "Taking ten minutes each Sunday to plan out your meals for the week, including sides, can seem like an added chore, but it will save you a load of stress and hassle in the week ahead," says Sally Kuzemchak, registered dietitian, author of *Cooking Light Dinnertime Survival Guide*, and the mother of two boys. Kuzemchak's advice includes batch cooking on the weekends and stocking up on convenient side dishes like frozen sweet potato French fries, instant brown rice or whole wheat couscous, canned beans, and frozen vegetables so meal preparation is fast and meals are well-rounded. Whatever your approach, a well-planned grocery list will keep your food purchases, budget, and trips to the store at a minimum.

Eating Right When Eating Out

Even during your best-planned weeks, you may find yourself unexpectedly at a restaurant, ordering from the local pizza joint, or breezing through the fast-food drive-through. "Sometimes it's just easier and less mess to hit the drive-through on the way home from practice," says Audrey, the mother of three athletes. "It would really help to know what to order."

According to a 2008 Gallup poll, the average American family eats dinner out one or more nights each week.[10] Eating out doesn't mean you have to give up on good nutrition. It's possible to have convenience and nutrition at the same time—you just need to know what to order. Here are my top tips for smart choices when eating out:

- Stick with lean protein options such as lean steak, beef fajitas, chicken breast, fish, and vegetarian options.
- Request that excess butter, oil, and cream sauces be left off.
- Ask for dressing and condiments to be served on the side.
- Ask to trade a high-fat side like French fries for veggies, salad, baked potato, or rice.
- Order milk instead of soda.
- Ask for whole-grain options, such as whole-wheat pasta or brown rice.
- Ask for your veggies steamed instead of sautéed or fried.
- Top salads with oil and vinegar. Salads with creamy dressings, cheese, and croutons are among the most fattening items on the menu.
- Share desserts and appetizers.

In addition to these tips, there are restaurants and menu items that are healthier than others, so try to pick these nutritious options when you go out to eat:

Italian: minestrone soup; pasta with marinara sauce; salad with vinaigrette dressing; seafood options

Chinese: hot and sour soup; steamed dishes; stir-fried veggies and meats; lettuce wraps; brown rice; seafood options; fresh fruit options

Japanese: edamame; sushi without tempura; sashimi; seaweed salad or a side salad with ginger dressing; hibachi meats, seafood, and veggies (request minimum oil use); brown rice; rice bowl meals; fresh fruit for dessert

Mexican: salsa, pico de gallo, and guacamole; grilled dishes with minimal cheese; fajitas (chicken, steak, shrimp); stuffed poblano peppers

Mediterranean: hummus; tabbouleh; baba ganouj; whole-wheat pitas; Greek salads with vinaigrette dressings; feta cheese; yogurt-based dips; seafood dishes; grilled dishes; gyros

Steakhouse: tomato/broth-based soups; broiled mushroom caps; grilled or broiled meat or seafood; baked potato or rice; steamed veggies; side salad; whole-grain bread

Pizza: salads; thin crust and/or whole-grain crust; veggie-style toppings; ham; grilled chicken; spaghetti or other pasta with marinara sauce

The goal for every young athlete is to eat balanced meals more often than not. How you accomplish this—whether you make meals at home, order in, or go out to eat—is up to you. You've got the tools to make a winning game plan—one that is a win-win for you, your athlete, and even your whole family.

Notes

1. The National Center on Addiction and Substance Abuse at Columbia University (CASAColumbia). "The importance of family dinner VIII." http://www.casacolumbia.org/addiction-research/reports/importance-of-family-dinners-2012.

2. Rampersaud GC, Benefits of breakfast for children and adolescents: Update and recommendations for practitioners. *Am J Lifestyle Med.* 3(2009): 86–103.
3. Cook E and Dunifon R. "Do family meals really make a difference?" Parenting in Context, Cornell University College of Human Ecology. http://www .human.cornell.edu/pam/outreach/upload/Family-Mealtimes-2.pdf.
4. Diehl K, Thiel A, Zipfel S, Mayer J, Litaker DG, and Schneider S. "How healthy is the behavior of young athletes? A systematic literature review and meta-analyses." *J Sports Sci Med.* 11 (2012): 201–220.
5. U.S. Department of Agriculture. ChooseMyPlate.gov Website. Washington, DC.
6. Morford KS. *Best Lunch Box Ever: Ideas and Recipes for School Lunches Kids Will Love.* San Francisco: Chronicle Books, 2013.
7. Castle JL and Jacobsen MT. *Fearless Feeding: How to Raise Healthy Eaters from High Chair to High School.* New York: Jossey-Bass, 2013.
8. The Huffington Post. "Cooking survey reveals that 28% of Americans can't cook." http://www.huffingtonpost.com/2011/09/09/cooking-survey_n _955600.html.
9. Joseph N. "42% of parents teach their kids how to cook in order to teach them a useful life skill." Researchscape. http://www.researchscape.com/ health/cooking-with-children-survey.
10. Saad L. "Restaurant dining mostly holding up despite recession." Gallup. http://www.gallup.com/poll/113617/restaurant-dining-mostly-holding -despite-recession.aspx.

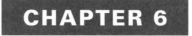

CHAPTER 6

Take a Time Out—Top Off with Snacks

It's not about how much you put into your body, it's about what you put into your body. I learned that by fueling my body properly, I train and perform much better than when I eat too much or too little.
—Nim Shapira, 2008 and 2012 Olympic swimmer

"That is the worst possible snack you could be eating right now," I overheard a swim coach say to a very young boy who was getting ready for a daylong meet. He turned around and repeated this statement to the child's dad: "You know, that's the worst thing he could be eating right now."

I admit it—I have a soft spot for coaches who openly guide their athletes and parents with healthy eating advice. Many young athletes are eating the worst snacks and are clueless when it comes to what a healthy snack is and when to eat it.

There is absolutely nothing wrong with snacks or snacking. In fact, I'm an advocate of snacks, especially for the growing athlete. Yet I know that snacks cause many parents to fret; they question whether snacking is good for their child, and which snacks are best. And it's true: many athletes just don't get it and repeatedly choose the wrong snack for athletic performance and overall health. This drives parents and coaches nuts.

While snacks can be a good source of nutrition for kids, there's a dark side to snacking that threatens to derail health, especially in the sports arena.

Take Davis, for example. A 10-year-old soccer player, he ate donuts and drank a juice box as a halftime pick-me-up, and chips and packaged cookies in celebration of every game—whether he played or not (and even if he did play, he didn't play for the whole hour). Twelve-year-old Jessica munched on candy between her swimming events at weekend meets, and 9-year-old Sam finished off his Saturday morning hockey practice with a run through the local donut shop. Seventeen-year-old Tyler munched all night long on snack food, the result of being under-fueled with snacks during his daily football training. And 14-year-old Jenny just loved sweets and junk food; she always chose chips, ice cream, and cookies for her snacks. Snacks like these can be problematic for the young athlete. In fact, they can single-handedly wipe out any health benefits provided by sports participation and healthy meals.

What is the point of a snack for the athlete anyway? And if snacks are so important, how can you get your athlete to eat the right stuff? This chapter explores why and when snacks are needed, who needs them (one answer: not the 8-year-old who has a 1-hour practice), and which snacks fit the bill for the young athlete. I'll offer good options for packaged snacks, as well as for whole and natural-food snacks, and give you some easy-to-make recipes for granola, smoothies, and what I call energy bites.

Snacking for Success

Athletes have a plethora of snacking options at their fingertips, although that fact comes with some pros and cons. If you do a "snack run" at the grocery store, you will find entire aisles filled with options such as cookies, crackers, and chips. You can find healthy versions too, such as individually packaged nuts, cereals, yogurts, and whole fruit and veggies. With every option, you'll want to consider ease of eating, ease of storage, digestibility, and, ultimately, the quality of fuel the snack provides.

Snacking is a big part of kids' and teen's daily eating. Up to 25% of daily calories consumed by children come from snacks and teens consume 26% of their calories from them.[1] The upside of this is that snacks can increase athletes' intake of nutrients such as protein, folate, vitamin C, magnesium, iron, potassium, and fiber. The downside is that they tend to deliver more calories in the form of sugar and unhealthy fats, and potentially contribute to extra weight and poor health.[2]

What this means is that you have the difficult job of keeping snacks on the straight and narrow for your athlete, making sure they scream "healthy" and help athletic performance, rather than detract from it. The hardest part is that kids often snack independently, freely, and someplace where you aren't, which presents its own set of challenges.

While unhealthy snacks always have tempted the taste buds of young athletes, and probably always will, learning how to navigate snack food options will help them succeed in playing their sport. Otherwise, it is just too easy for them to go for the chocolate chip muffin or the cookie. It won't be easy for you to advise your young athletes on snacking unless you understand what drives their choices. Let's look at the reasons young athletes pick the snacks they do.

The Role of Taste

Taste is a big driver for food choice among kids and teens.[3] If food doesn't taste good, or even *look like* it will taste good, they won't eat it. Food manufacturers understand this, dumping loads of money into research to develop irresistible flavors. You need to be just as savvy as the manufacturers are, and make sure that your food tastes and looks good so you'll have a better chance at having your young athletes eat what you serve or pack for practices and competitions.

Understanding Hunger

When athletes are hungry, they want to eat! Now! This urgent hunger is physiological, as hunger and appetite are by-products of intense exercise. Some sports, such as swimming, rowing, and distance running, make athletes hungrier than others. Parents can curtail the fierceness of physiological hunger by staying ahead of it with nutritious meals and snacks served on a schedule, as outlined in Chapter 5 (see page 124). The problem is that some athletes, rather than experiencing true physical hunger, may think they are hungry (I call this head hunger), and this can lead to overeating.

The good news is that you can help your athletes recognize true physical hunger as the primary cue for eating, and have good food ready for them when hunger rears its ugly head after they exercise. Point out and explain head hunger; for example, it's when your athletes ask for food an hour after a full meal when it's unlikely that they're physiologically hungry. Staying on track with your meal and snack structure will help keep your athletes fueled and eating when they really need food.

Question Advertising and the Media

Advertising sells food, and many advertised foods are not good choices for the growing athlete. Young athletes are saturated with advertising; it is on every medium that young people use—mobile phones, TV, and computer laptops—and even on billboards at sporting venues. This advertising bombardment triggers a desire to eat because young athletes' developmental stages make them susceptible to advertising's message. The food ads that kids and teens see really do influence their purchases and ultimately their food preferences.[4]

While you cannot eliminate advertising from your athletes' lives, you can help them understand it. For example, when Olympic and professional athletes appear in commercials eating fast food and drinking sodas, challenge your athletes by questioning the reality of these representations: Do Olympians truly eat fast food to sustain their performance? Not likely! Help your athletes become media-literate by talking about marketing messages. Question the intent behind advertising (which is to get your athletes to buy and to become loyal customers). Talk about the reality of the message, and weigh the consequences of eating junk food on health and performance. Encourage skepticism: it's healthy to doubt and question, especially when it comes to advertised food products that target athletes.

Available Snacks Are the Ones Kids Eat

Convenience also drives what athletes choose to eat. Fast food, pantry snacks, and what's in the fridge and at the concession stand are what athletes are tempted to eat. The easier a snack is to grab and eat, the more likely your athletes will devour it. This can work in your favor when you have nutritious snacks on hand. Cut up fruit and put it out on the counter at home. Make snacks that are fast and easy to eat, at home, in the cooler, and at sporting events. For example, make sandwiches, cut them into squares, and wrap them in tin foil. Voila! They become a snack rather than a lunch staple. Bite-size servings of finger food and small portions (think snack bags of gorp) encourage moderate consumption, while large bags of chips or popcorn encourage grazing and overeating. Remember, if your young athletes are like most, they eat a lot of snacks every day, so do your best to make healthy options easy and accessible.

Addressing the Pack Mentality

Kids are pack animals. They are tuned into their friends—what they are doing, wearing, and eating. Young athletes want to be part of the group and will adopt behaviors, even about food and eating, that keep them in the loop. If Jessica is munching on candy between swim events, her peers are probably doing the same.

To change the pack mentality, you have to address the pack. Encourage a team policy about proper snack foods, and plan concession food that supports healthy snacking and gets the whole group into a healthy eating routine.

Some stubborn athletes may still choose unhealthy foods out of habit or a misguided loyalty to what "everyone else" is doing. You may have to take the "village" approach, using other parents, the coaching staff, and celebrity role models who get the nutrition approach right to help influence your teen. I discuss how to do this in Chapter 7 and how to set healthy policies about food and sports in Chapter 10.

A lot of learning about food and eating takes place during childhood and adolescence, and mistakes are par for the course. Table 6-1 lists common snacking dilemmas among young athletes and what to do about them.

Why Should Athletes Snack?

There are three main reasons young athletes should eat well-planned snacks: to keep their appetites satisfied so that they can avoid overeating later; to provide any nutrients that aren't covered by meals; and to fuel the body for exercise. When you keep these reasons in mind, it becomes easy

Table 6-1 Common Snacking Dilemmas and Solutions

Snacking Dilemma	What It Looks Like	Solution
Starving after school	After school, your athlete is "about to die" if he or she doesn't eat. There may be evidence of inadequate eating earlier in the day: leftovers in lunchbox, or incomplete breakfast consumption.	Front-load the day with nutrition. Make sure a hearty breakfast is on board including a protein source. Encourage a balanced and nutritious lunch, either from school or packed from home, and include a morning snack if needed.
Never full enough ("always hungry")	This can be due to not eating enough food at meals, eating unhealthy items, or being out of touch with real hunger.	Plan a regular meal and snack schedule to occur every 3 to 4 hours; check to make sure food items are wholesome, nutritious, and satisfying; help your athlete tune into physical hunger versus head hunger (thinking that you're hungry).
Grazes or nibbles all day	This is more of an eating style or eating personality.	Offer high-nutrient snacks and boost meals with extra nutritious options so that it's easy for the athlete to meet calorie and nutrient needs.
Loves junk food	If unhealthy snack items are readily available and there are no limits around eating them, many athletes will opt for them.	Reign in junk food to one or two items per day. Hold the line on this boundary. Allow athlete to choose *which* junk foods he or she will eat that day.

to find suitable snacks, and when strategically placed between meals or around athletic practices or events, snacks can keep your athlete's appetite on an even keel and tame crazy hunger surges.

Your athlete's appetite will match what's going on with his or her growth and physical changes. Wanting to eat is not a bad thing—hunger is the natural signal for the body to seek what it needs. But hunger can turn into an out-of-control feeling, leading your athlete to eat anything and everything in sight. The roots of this problem are in the timing and content of meals. For example, if meals and snacks are eaten on an erratic schedule or the time intervals between them are long, an athlete may well become hungry.

Likewise, meals that aren't sufficiently nutritious and that provide too few calories can increase hunger. The effects of one inadequate meal can be corrected by eating more at the next meal, but if this up-and-down eating becomes a pattern, mental and physical feelings of hunger can get out of hand and grow into an unhealthy drive to eat too much or the wrong things between meals. The more erratic your meal schedule is, the more erratic and unpredictable your athlete's hunger and appetite may be. The danger, of course, is that snacks will become the answer to your athlete's hunger, when it should be the other way around—meals are the primary fuel, and snacks top off the tank. The antidote to this problem is to deliver meals and snacks on a predictable schedule.

Protein helps satiate the appetite, according to research conducted at the University of Missouri. Study participants who ate a high-protein snack delayed their requests for subsequent meals because they felt full longer.[5] Another study in children showed that when certain foods were paired, for example vegetables and cheese, children ate 72% fewer calories before becoming full. Researchers found that the addition of protein (cheese, in this case) was more satisfying to the appetite and contributed to fullness and a lower calorie intake.[6]

Snacks should be nutrient-rich, providing high levels of nutrients within a reasonable amount of calories. A good example of a nutrient-rich snack item is Greek yogurt. It's rich in protein, calcium, vitamin D, potassium, and phosphorus, and has a reasonable amount of calories (about 140 per 6 to 8 ounces [177 to 237 mL]). Compare this to potato chips, which provide your athlete saturated fat, some salt, and 150 calories—all with just 1 ounce (28 g), or 10 chips. Comparing the nutritional quality of various snacks can be an eye-opening experience.

Nutrient-rich snacks help your athletes get closer to their daily nutritional requirements for growth, development, and performance. These snacks can do a good job of closing the gap between what your athletes have eaten earlier in the day and what remains for them to eat in order to meet their nutritional needs. For example, if they skip their morning dairy product, you know you can help them make it up at snack time with yogurt, cheese, or a glass of milk. If they've sailed through breakfast and lunch without fruits and veggies, you can include both in a smoothie that you make for their afternoon snack.

Lastly, but most importantly for the athlete, snacks help ready the body for exercise and speed recovery from intense bouts of it. Sports nutritionists call this *nutrient timing*. Nutrient timing—when to eat for optimal performance and recovery—is especially important for the serious young athlete. Timing the intake of food has the power to improve performance and build muscle, both of which help athletes get better at their sports. For a recap on carbohydrate and protein for recovery snacks, go back to Chapter 2 (page 54). Table 6-2 offers healthy snack ideas based on the needs of training and competition.

Table 6-2 Healthy Snack Options for Training and Competition

Everyday Training Snack	Pre-Competition or Workout*	Post-Competition or Workout*
1 cup (56 g) oatmeal squares cereal + ½ cup (119 mL) milk	½ cup (28 g) dry cereal	1 cup (237 mL) chocolate milk
1 slice (1 oz or 28 g) whole wheat toast + 1 tablespoon (11 g) peanut butter	Banana	1–2 tablespoons (11 to 22 g) peanut butter + 4 whole grain crackers
½ cup (74 g) fresh blueberries + 1 cup (237 mL) low fat yogurt	Small box (14 g) of raisins	6 ounces (164 mL) Greek yogurt
6 whole wheat crackers (28 g) + 1½ ounces (42 g) cheese	4–6 (19 to 28 g) whole wheat crackers	2 (56 g) mozzarella cheese sticks
1 mini-bagel (26 g) with 1 oz (28 g) deli ham and 1 oz (28 g) deli cheese	1 mini-bagel (26 g) with 1 tablespoon (14.5 g) of cream cheese	1 oz (28 g) turkey wrapped around a cheese stick (28 g) with 2–4 (9 to 19 g) whole wheat crackers
1 medium (173 g) baked potato with ⅓ cup (38 g) shredded cheese and 2 tablespoons (36 g) salsa	Small (1.5 oz or 43 g) bag of pita chips	1/3 cup (45 g) mixed nuts and 1 oz (28 g) dark chocolate bits
1 tablespoon (11 g) nut butter and 1 tablespoon (20 g) jam on 1 slice (1 oz or 28 g) of whole grain bread	Small bag (1 oz or 28 g) of pretzels	Peanut butter packet (2 tablespoons or 22 g) + 10 pretzel twists (60 g)
½ English muffin (29 g) pizza with 2 tablespoons (31 g) tomato sauce, 2 tablespoons (22 g) mozzarella cheese, and turkey pepperoni (15 g)	1/2 cup (61 g) of granola	2-1oz (56 g) yogurt sticks
Smoothie: ½ cup (75 g) frozen strawberries + ½ banana + ½ cup (119 mL) milk and ½ cup (119 mL) vanilla yogurt	4 ounces (119 mL) of yogurt	12 oz (355 mL) packaged smoothie drink (freeze ahead so it will defrost during practice)

*For workouts and competition lasting longer than 1 hour.

Who Gets a Snack?

Not everyone should get a snack when they exercise, although our present sports-snacking practices might lead you to believe otherwise. It's a mistake to offer young kids unneeded snacks at practices and games. All athletes can have one or two snacks a day, but a child doesn't get a pass for more snacks just because he or she runs around the field. Remember Davis, the boy who got snacks both at halftime and after his soccer game? This was too much food. Such snacks end up canceling out the benefits of exercise and often contribute to excessive calorie intake. When this happens, kids also get the wrong message about the role of snacks and exercise. They perceive snacks as a reward for activity. Rather, kids should learn to associate snacks—healthy, nutrient-rich snacks, not treats—with fuel for exercise.

Time Out!

For athletes involved in recreational sports and kids exercising for under an hour, no snack is needed before, during, or after game time. Start the day with a nutritious meal and proceed with regular meals and one to two snacks. If your child wants an additional snack, make it fruit or veggies. This will add nutrition to your child's day.

Because teens tend to exercise longer and perhaps with more intensity, they typically need a healthy snack before exercise to top off their tank with fuel. Tyler, who snacked all night long, could have overcome his urges to eat nonstop by getting some pre- and post-exercise fuel on board. Not only would this have helped his performance and recovery, it would've satisfied his appetite so that he wouldn't snack so late. Remember, teens need a post-exercise snack with protein and carbs to speed up the muscle-recovery process and help reload the muscles with glycogen when they participate in intense exercise bouts. These snacks help teen athletes get ready for their next exercise session.

Time Out!

For teens exercising for over an hour, provide a carbohydrate-based snack 30 minutes to 1 hour prior to exercising, as outlined in Chapter 5. Within 45 minutes after exercising, they should eat a combination snack that includes protein and carbohydrate. See Table 6-2 for ideas.

Healthy Snacks Rule!

From homemade to whole natural foods, there are endless options for healthy snacks. You should know about good options for packaged snacks, whole-food snacks, and do-it-yourself snacks (homemade) so that you have a variety to choose from based on your available time and skills in the kitchen. Before we get into which foods are good snack options, let's review how to combine nutrients to best suit your athlete's needs.

The Best Snacks

The best snacks for athletes showcase a blend of macronutrients, especially carbs and protein. Making sure a source of protein is included automatically morphs a snack from a lackluster offering to a "power snack." When you think about selecting foods to make a smart snack for your athlete, first think *carb + protein or fat.* Then think *mini-meal.* This approach to creating a snack helps keep your athletes' appetite satisfied, better answers their nutrient needs, and supplies the nutrients they require to both prepare before and recover after exercise.

How to Make a Power Snack

1.   *Choose a carb.* Select whole-grain crackers, cereal, bread, pretzels, bagel, English muffin, pasta, rice, waffle, pancake, dried fruit, 100% juice, raw veggies, or fresh fruit.

2.   *Add protein.* Choose milk, egg, yogurt, cheese, cottage cheese, deli meat, peanut butter, nuts (like almonds, peanuts, cashews or pistachios), seeds, hummus, or beans.

3.   *Or add fat.* Opt for olive oil, avocado, butter, olives, nuts, seeds, cheese, or whole milk (also contains protein). Remember that many foods such as cheese and yogurt, meats, and nuts have fat built into them.

4.   *Put your mini-meal together.* Once you decide on your food combination, check your portion sizes using the portion guide in Table 5-1. Remember, some foods already have protein, carbs, and fat naturally built in, such as yogurt, other dairy products, and granola bars with added protein. Check out these healthy-snack examples: a milk-and-fruit blended smoothie; a hard-boiled egg and raw veggies; cheese and crackers; dry cereal and dried fruit; pretzels and hummus; yogurt and fruit; deli meat and bread; peanut butter and a banana.

Now that you know how to build a substantial, satisfying snack, let's go through your options from the grocery store and some items you can make at home.

A Word about Packaged Snacks

Before you pick up the cheesy square crackers, fishy shapes, or the chocolate-coated granola bar, you need to be aware of the pitfalls inherent with packaged snacks.

Understanding the Ingredient List. The ingredient list is your clue to what's really inside that snack. Watch out for chemicals and unidentifiable ingredients. If you can't pronounce it and you don't know what it is, be skeptical. Mystery ingredients should alert you to additives, colors, artificial sweeteners, and other undesirable ingredients. Think twice before purchasing such items; a healthy athlete's diet contains as few unknown ingredients as possible. Remember that the first item on the ingredient list is the product's most prominent ingredient, and the others follow in the order of their prominence in the product. The first three ingredients should be wholesome items such as whole wheat, oats, or peanuts, rather than things you want to minimize in your athlete's diet, such as sugar.

A Nutrition Checklist. Look at the proportion of nutrients in each serving your athlete will be eating from a particular snack. You can find this on the Nutrition Facts label. Keep the following in mind:

Calories. In general, snacks should contain 150 to 250 calories per serving. More than that and it's not a "snack."

Added sugar. Keep added sugar to less than 9 grams per serving. Added sugar is high fructose corn syrup (HFCS), maple syrup, table sugar, and more. Lactose or fructose, the natural sugars found in dairy products and fruit, do not qualify as "added."

Total fat. Aim for less than 30% of calories per serving from total fat. Ideally, we should be eating products that have more mono- and poly-unsaturated fats than saturated and trans-fats.

Fiber. Shoot for 5 grams of fiber or more per serving. Many snacks made from whole grains are good sources of fiber.

Sodium. Keep it as low as you can, targeting less than 240 milligrams per serving or 10% of the Daily Value (DV).

Daily Value. Aim for the fiber, calcium, iron, and vitamins A and C in the product to contribute 10% or more of the DV for each.

Good packaged snack options include granola bars with mostly whole ingredients and limited sugar (nix the candy-coated bars); granola bars with up to 10 grams of protein per serving; trail mixes that include nuts; raisins and other individually packaged dried fruit; whole-grain cereal boxes; boxed milk, chocolate milk, and soymilk; packaged whole-grain oatmeal (just add water or milk); whole-grain crackers with nut butter or cheese; and applesauce and other pureed fruits and vegetable blends.

Some snacks are not good for the young athlete. Table 6-3 lists 10 of the worst snacks for your athlete.

Table 6-3 10 of the Worst Snacks for Athletes

Snack	Reason
Candy bars	High sugar elevates blood sugar and may lead to a crash (low blood sugar episode); high fat content slows digestion and may cause stomach cramps
Sugary candy	High sugar content leads to quick elevation of blood sugar; may experience a reactive low blood sugar; lack of other nutrients
Soda	No nutrients; high sugar content; can be filling and cause gassiness
Chips such as tortilla, potato, corn	High fat and salt content, low nutrients
Candy-coated granola bars	Nutrient profile may be similar to that of a candy bar
Sweet desserts such as donuts, cupcakes, and cookies	High in sugar, fat, and calorie content
Greasy frozen pizza bites and hand-held "pocket" sandwiches	High fat, processed, and low in nutrients; check the label for healthy options
Ice cream and other frozen dairy based treats; milkshakes	High sugar and fat content; should be reserved for special occasions
French fries	High fat and salt content; about 10 calories per fry
Juice boxes	Typically contain added sugar; look for 100% juice and keep portions to 8–12 (237 to 355 mL) ounces maximum per day

Whole Food Snacks

Unadulterated and pure in form, these snacks are generally healthy and nutritious. Many just need a quick wash and minimal prep. Bananas, grapes (frozen grapes are a good stand-in for candy), apples, berries, stone fruits like peaches and nectarines, and all kinds of dried fruit make excellent, carb-rich snacks. Try all-fruit leathers, also. Carrots, snap peas, and red peppers are also great carb-based snacks; add the power of protein with some hummus or cheese. Nuts are an excellent source of protein and healthy fats. Bag them in snack bags or buy them packaged in 1-ounce (28 g) portions. Guacamole (mashed avocado), a healthy fat, can be bought in single-serve packs and paired with whole-grain tortilla or other whole-grain chips. Edamame in the shell and hard-boiled eggs make an excellent protein addition to any snack.

Do-It-Yourself (DIY) Snacks

Muffins, granola, roasted beans, trail mix, breakfast cookies, and what I call pucks and energy bites can all be made at home in your kitchen, where you control the amounts of sugar and additives (see the next section for recipes). Better yet, many of these can be made and frozen, ready to pull out of the freezer as needed. The best thing about DIY snacks is knowing what they contain, and knowing you're adding to the overall nutrition of your athlete.

Preventing Snack Spoilage

Make sure you either properly cool snacks that can spoil or pack nutritious snacks that don't require refrigeration. Some snacks—yogurt, deli meat sandwiches, hummus and other dips—need to be packed on ice to prevent bacterial contamination and spoilage. While fruit, veggies, and drinks don't require cooling, they often taste better and go down easier when they are cold. Food items that can safely be tossed into the duffle bag include nuts and nut butters, dried fruit, dry cereal, beef jerky, pretzels, seeds, and Fig Newton cookies.

Snack Recipes for the Athlete

The easiest way to ensure that your young athlete will be eating nutritious snacks is to use the different snack resources outlined above to guarantee healthy snacking—it's what I do for my own athletes. From prepackaged to whole-food combos and homemade versions, you have several options to optimize what your athlete snacks on. Here are some healthy DIY recipes you can make now and freeze for later.

Oatmeal, Peanut Butter Chip, and Banana Pucks

2 eggs

3 ripe bananas, mashed

1 tablespoon (15 mL) vanilla

1 tablespoon (15 mL) baking powder

3 cups (280 g) oatmeal

¼ cup (48 g) sugar

½ cup (120 g) peanut butter chips

1 cup (237 mL) low fat milk

2 tablespoons (30 mL) chia seeds (optional)

Preheat oven to 375ºF. Coat a 12-cup muffin tin with nonstick cooking spray. Combine all ingredients in a large bowl, mixing until thoroughly combined. Fill each well in the tin to the top with the oatmeal mixture. Bake for 18 to 20 minutes or until slightly browned on top and firm to the touch. Cool on a rack completely.

Homemade Chewy Sweet and Buttery Granola

3 cups (240 g) rolled oats

¼ cup (59 mL) canola oil

⅓ cup (63 g) packed light brown sugar

½ teaspoon (2.5 mL) cinnamon

¼ teaspoon (1.25 mL) kosher salt

¼ cup (59 mL) honey

1 teaspoon (5 mL) butter extract

½ cup (60 g) coarse chopped cashews (optional)

Heat the oil in a large skillet over medium heat. Add oats and stir until they are brown and crisp, about 5 to 10 minutes. Take off the heat and stir in the brown sugar, cinnamon, salt, honey and butter extract, stirring constantly, coating the oats for about 5 minutes. Pour the mixture onto a cookie sheet to cool. After it is cooled, mix in chopped cashews. Store in an airtight container or freeze.

Salt and Pepper Roasted Chickpeas

1 (29-ounce [822-g]) can chickpeas, rinsed, drained, and patted dry

2 tablespoons (30 mL) olive oil

1 teaspoon (5 mL) kosher salt

½ teaspoon 2.5 mL mL) black pepper

Preheat oven to 450ºF. In a bowl, toss together the chickpeas, olive oil, salt, and pepper. Spread on a baking sheet and roast for 25 to 35 minutes, until brown and crunchy.

Homestyle Trail Mix

1, 14.5 ounce- box of whole-grain cereal squares (mini-wheats, oatmeal squares, plain Cheerios)

1, 12 ounce-bag butter-flavored pretzel squares

2 cups (320 g) dried raisins

2 cups (336 g) lightly salted peanuts

1, 11 ounce-bag (312 g) M & M's candy

Mix all ingredients in a large bowl until thoroughly combined. Divide into snack bags, placing about ½ cup (80 to 90 g) of mix into each.

Oat Flax and Raisin Breakfast Cookies

2 sticks of salted butter, softened (224 g)

¾ cup (144 g) lightly packed brown sugar

1 teaspoon (5 mL) vanilla extract

1 teaspoon (5 mL) cinnamon

1½ cups (120 g) rolled oats

1 cup (80 g) quick-cooking oats

2 eggs

½ cup applesauce (128 g)

2 cups (240 g) whole wheat flour

1 cup (104 g) ground flaxseed

1 teaspoon (5 mL) baking soda

1¼ cups (200 g) raisins

Preheat oven to 375°F. In a large mixing bowl, combine the butter, sugar, vanilla, and cinnamon until smooth. Add the oats, mixing well after each type. Add eggs and applesauce, mixing well after each addition. Add flour, flax, baking soda, and raisins, mixing well. Dough will be stiff. Line a baking sheet with parchment paper. Use a ¼ cup measure to shape and portion cookies; place the cookie disks on the sheet, evenly spaced. Press slightly to flatten. Bake for 10 to 12 minutes or until browned on the edges. Let cool on the baking sheet before moving to a wired cooling rack. Makes 24 cookies.

Peanut Butter Chocolate Chip Energy Bites

⅔ cup (118 g) peanut butter

1 cup (80 g) old-fashioned oats

½ cup (52 g) ground flaxseed

½ cup (120 g) chocolate chips

⅓ cup (78 mL) maple syrup

½ teaspoon (2.5 mL) cinnamon

1 tablespoon (15 mL) chia seeds

Place all the ingredients in a mixing bowl and mix together with clean hands until thoroughly combined. Cover and refrigerate for 30 minutes or until firm and not sticky. Roll into balls 1 inch (2.5 cm) in diameter using a small scoop or spoon. Store in an airtight container for 3 days on the counter, 1 week in the fridge, or 1 month in the freezer.

Rock the House Smoothie

½ cup (119 mL) plain Greek yogurt

1 cup (165 g) frozen mango

½ cup (119 mL) orange juice

A drizzle of honey

In a blender, combine the juice, yogurt, frozen fruit, and honey. Blend on high until completely blended and smooth.

Notes

1. U.S. Department of Agriculture and U.S. Department of Health and Human Services. *"Dietary Guidelines for Americans, 2015."* Available at: http://www.health.gov/dietaryguidelines/2015-scientific-report/PDFs/Scientific-Report-of-the-2015-Dietary-Guidelines-Advisory-Committee.pdf

2. Larson N and Story M. "A review of snacking patterns among children and adolescents: what are the implications of snacking for weight status?" *Child Obes.* 9 (2013):104–115.

3. Scaglioni S, Arrizza C, Vecchi F, and Tedeschi S. "Determinants of children's eating behaviour." *Am J Clin Nutr.* 94 (2011): 2006s–2011s.

4. Harris JL, Pomeranz JL, Lobstein T, and Brownell KD. "A crisis in the marketplace: how food marketing contributes to childhood obesity and what can be done." *Annu Rev Pub Health.* 30 (2009): 211–225.

5. Leidy HJ and Campbell WW. "The effect of eating frequency on appetite control and food intake: brief synopsis of controlled feeding studies." *J Nutr.* 141 (2011):154–157.

6. Wansink B, Shimizu M, and Brumberg A. "Association of nutrient-dense snack combinations with calories and vegetable intake." *Pediatrics.* 131 (2013):22–29.

CHAPTER 7

Foul Play—Supplements and Performance Aids

If it works, it's probably banned. If it's not banned, it's probably useless.
—Ron Maughan, sports nutrition scientist and member of the
International Olympic Committee Expert Panel on Nutrition

David was a sophomore rower who was working hard over
the summer to lower his erg score (the time it takes a rower
to cover a set distance on an ergometer or rowing machine),
rowing every day and doing strength training. "He wants to
take a dietary supplement containing branched-chain amino
acids [BCAAs]," said his mom, Janet. "He thinks this will help
his muscles recover and prevent the buildup of lactic acid [a
by-product of exercise that builds up in muscle and blood,
causing temporary muscle soreness and fatigue]. I'm not
certain if this supplement is helpful, whether it's necessary,
or whether it could be harmful."

Janet was fortunate that her son came to her with his request. Like
many parents, she was worried, and her fear and skepticism were warranted. Unfortunately, some young athletes don't discuss the topic of supplements with their parents. They just start taking them, leaving their

parents and coaches in the dark. If you have a young athlete, you can't afford to be naive about supplements.

Many studies have been done on supplements, but most of them focus on adults; there are few supplement studies in teens, and there has been only scant research on the effects of supplements on children. Yet supplement use by young athletes is growing by leaps and bounds. Presently, about 5% of middle school and high school students use anabolic steroids, an illegal supplement used to build muscle.[1] More than a third of boys and a fifth of girls use protein powders to enhance muscle, and 10% use nonsteroid anabolic aids like creatine to improve athletic performance.[2]

Even the illegal use of human growth hormone (HGH), a substance traditionally used to treat a variety of medical conditions, including short stature in children, is on the upswing in young athletes. In a 2014 survey sponsored by MetLife Foundation called the Partnership Attitude Tracking Study (PATS), 11% of teens in the ninth to twelfth grades reported using HGH without a prescription, more than twice the rates found in 2012. This survey also found that the use of steroids has increased by 2% since 2009.[3] It's clear that teens are increasingly interested in and are using legal and illegal substances to enhance their physical performance and appearance. Even if your athlete isn't using them, he or she very likely knows about supplements, hears the hype, and has questions. You owe it to your athlete to be knowledgeable about these substances.

Although I present a lot of technical terminology in this chapter, I also provide practical advice and tables you can refer to when you need them. My goal is to help you appreciate the variety of supplements available to your athlete, their effect on his or her performance, and the potential dangers. Supplements are the "bad influence" you don't want your kid hanging out with. However, simply forbidding the use of supplements may make them more attractive. We need to be savvy and aware so that we can fully educate our young athletes and guide them as potential experiences come their way.

The Scoop on Supplements

Did you know that dietary supplements, including weight-loss products, vitamin and mineral supplements, and similar substances, are some of the top-selling products in the United States? Our nation's love affair with the "quick fix" makes diet pills, muscle builders, and pain-free exercise sexy and seductive. In 2012, dietary supplements raked in $32 billion. And there doesn't appear to be a ceiling to their popularity; the industry is projected to grow to $60 billion by 2021, as reported in *Forbes* magazine.[4] Furthermore, global industry analysis predicts the market for sports nutrition products alone will grow to over $6 billion by 2018.[5]

Supplements, Defined

While performance-enhancing agents vary in type and purpose, they are generally used for building or strengthening muscle, quickening recovery after exercise, assisting or strengthening the immune system, and helping to trim body fat. Beverages such as sports drinks are not considered supplements, but energy drinks fall within the category due to some of their ingredients, such as herbal preparations and caffeine.

What Is a Performance-Enhancing Supplement?

Performance-enhancing supplements may be ergogenic aids—that is, supplements designed to increase strength, power, speed, or endurance. Or they may alter body weight or body composition (muscle and fat), or change behavior, alertness, and the perception of pain.

Performance-enhancing supplements may include the following:

Prescription medications taken in doses beyond prescribed amounts or when they're not needed, such as asthma inhalers when breathing spasms aren't present

Weight-control agents such as stimulants, diet pills, diuretics, or laxatives, which athletes in certain sports use to "make weight" (qualify for competition by coming in under a certain set weight limit)

Weight-gain agents such as protein powders, used to pack on more muscle

Oxygen-carrying-capacity agents, such as erythropoietin or transfusions (blood doping), which deliver more oxygen to the muscles

Nutrients such as vitamins or herbal preparations, taken at extra-high doses for a health or athletic benefit (beyond what is normally required)

Most of the research available on young athletes' experience with supplements tells us whether they take them and which ones they are using. For example, the National Health Interview Survey found that 94.5% of kids and teens used multivitamin supplements, 43% used fish oil, 34% used creatine, and 26% used fiber supplements.[6] In teens alone, 24% to 29% took performance-enhancing supplements, and this rate increased as involvement in sports and physical activity increased.[7] What the research doesn't tell us is how supplements behave in the young athlete's body, and this is concerning.

"I see athletes making the mistake of taking a supplement or ergogenic aid without really understanding how it may affect their body," says Heather Mangieri, a sports dietitian and owner of Nutrition CheckUp in Pittsburgh, Pennsylvania. "They may feel an energy drink or other central nervous system stimulant will help them feel more energized without realizing the product will likely disrupt their sleep habits. They easily end up in a vicious cycle of low energy, energy drink, trouble sleeping and continue to repeat this pattern day after day."

Regulating Supplements

Whether you're a newbie or are wise to this corner of the sports world, understanding how supplements are regulated will help you appreciate why and how they've become so popular. Dietary supplements are a food subcategory and as such are regulated by the U.S. Food and Drug Administration (FDA), along with the Federal Trade Commission (FTC). These organizations define supplements more broadly, as follows:

A product (other than tobacco) that is intended to supplement the diet, containing one or more of the following dietary ingredients: a vitamin, a mineral, an herb or other botanical, an amino acid, a dietary substance for use by man to supplement the diet by increasing the total daily intake, or a concentrate, metabolite, constituent, extract, or combinations of these ingredients.

Intended for ingestion in pill, capsule, tablet, or liquid form.

Not represented for use as a conventional food or as the sole item of a meal or diet.

Labeled as a "dietary supplement."[8]

The FDA regulates the safety, claims, and labeling of both finished dietary supplement products and ingredients, while the FTC regulates their advertising and marketing. The Dietary Supplement Health and Education Act of 1994 (DSHEA; see box) is the primary legislation that defines and governs dietary supplements in the United States. It places dietary supplements under the broad umbrella of "foods," not drugs, and requires every supplement to be labeled a dietary supplement.

While this legislation was well intentioned in its conception and governing, my saying that the FDA regulates dietary supplements may mislead you into believing that they are safe and controlled by the government. Unfortunately, the regulation of dietary supplements has too many loopholes, including unsubstantiated claims of efficacy; possible contamination with illegal ingredients; easy accessibility, particularly to children and teens; and a reactive stance relying on consumer reporting—all of which I will cover later in this chapter.

As the young consumer is increasingly able to gain access and use supplements, the dangers and negative consequences become more concerning and apparent. I believe there should be more control over supplements by governing bodies, particularly for young athletes.

The Truth about Supplement Regulation

If a supplement contains an ingredient that existed prior to 1994, when the Dietary Supplement Health and Education Act was passed, the supplement is considered safe. This means that new combinations of previously approved ingredients can be created, marketed, and sold with the presumption of safety. The FDA does not have the authority to require safety testing prior to manufacturers' advertising and marketing supplements that contain previously approved ingredients.

If a *new* ingredient is introduced—one that did not exist prior to 1994—the product is considered unsafe unless proven otherwise, and manufacturers must perform safety and efficacy testing prior to releasing the product to market. All supplement manufacturers must ensure that claims about their products are accurate. However, the FDA does not conduct reviews before a product comes to market to determine if it is effective or safe; this is left to the manufacturer.

Once a product is on the market and available to consumers, the manufacturer, not the FDA, is responsible for ensuring the product's safety. Supplement manufacturers have been criticized for not investigating the potential side effects and safety of their products.

In the event that a supplement is suspected of being unsafe, ineffective, or including undeclared substances, the burden of proof rests with the FDA to remove it from the market.[9,10] In essence, the FDA relies on consumers to bring problematic supplements to its attention. Thus, this means that supplements can fly under the radar of regulatory scrutiny, while largely entering the market under the assumption of safety.

The Lure of Supplements

Males are more likely to use performance-enhancing supplements than females. However, females aren't immune to the promise of better, faster performance. Studies of usage vary; one study found that between 11% and 76% of females have tried or routinely take the performance-enhancing supplements creatine or caffeine.[11] The two biggest reasons young athletes want to take supplements are to build muscle (which usually means getting faster, stronger, and athletically better) and to improve their appearance—specifically, to look more lean and muscular.

Some experts believe that the high school sports culture encourages young athletes, especially boys, to use supplements. In a 2006 study, researchers suggested that high school sports provide an early introduction to legal performance-enhancing substances as a way to improve physical performance, and minimized the perception of risks associated with them.[12] Other studies have found that parents and coaches are pivotal in recommending the use of performance-enhancing substances.[13] My own experience has supported this; parents have told me they have encouraged their athletes to take a certain supplement to help them bulk up, increase speed, or lean out.

Young athletes are susceptible when it comes to supplements; they feel peer pressure, value reward over risk, and may fail to understand the long-term dangers or consequences associated with supplements. Some people point the finger at the behavior of sports idols and an attitude within our overall culture that suggests that success cannot be had without performance-enhancing substances.[14]

Finally, advertising and marketing that targets teen athletes may pique their interest and curiosity. Understanding why your athlete is interested in supplements is key to helping you deal with this issue, and I'll talk more about this later in this chapter. But first, you need a primer on supplements.

Supplements Used by Young Athletes

If I had a dollar for every supplement available on the market today, I wouldn't be a millionaire, but I'd have a nice little nest egg. There are many supplements out there, and they come and go. This alone makes it challenging—even confusing and intimidating—to stay on top of them. Thankfully, there are organizations that take care of tracking the important stuff for you, and I'll dig into those soon.

Some supplements come as single-ingredient products, such as creatine, while others combine several ingredients in one product, such as energy drinks.

Below I describe the most common supplements used by young athletes. Parents who want or need to deal with supplements should be curious about their ingredients and should use the resources listed later in the chapter to learn about their function, safety, and effectiveness (see box "Where Can I Find Reliable Information about Supplements?").

Creatine

Studies over the years have consistently found that teen athletes use supplemental creatine as a performance-enhancing substance. In smaller amounts, it is naturally found in foods such as beef, poultry, and fish. Studies in adults have shown that creatine increases power and force in short exercise bouts and increases athletic performance with repeated activity. There is less evidence available regarding their use in teens; however, more studies are being conducted in this area. For this reason and because of the unknown effects of creatine on the heart, kidneys, and reproductive organs in growing athletes, the American Academy of Pediatrics (AAP) and the American College of Sports Medicine (ACSM) advise against the use of creatine by athletes under the age of 18.[15] However, the International Society for Sports Nutrition (ISSN) outlines numerous conditions for the appropriate use of creatine in young elite athletes who have completed puberty.[16] Side effects of creatine may include weight gain; stomach problems, including diarrhea, nausea, gas, burping, and stomach pain; kidney problems; dehydration; and an irregular heartbeat.

Beta-Hydroxy-Beta-Methylbutyrate

Beta-hydroxy-beta-methylbutyrate (HMB), a by-product of the branched-chain amino acid (BCAA) leucine, is found naturally in foods such as catfish, citrus fruits, and breast milk. It limits the breakdown of protein and cell damage after intense exercise, which may lead to quicker recovery, a lower requirement for rest between intensive exercise sessions, and more lean muscle and strength.[17,18] Teens are attracted to this supplement for its muscle-building, appearance-enhancing features. The typical dose is 1.5 to 3 grams per day; higher doses haven't shown any additional benefit. In fact, HMB doesn't seem to offer much benefit at all to the trained athlete because the muscles are already adapted to exercise. Its optimal role appears to be during the start of training, when muscles are adapting to exercise, as demonstrated in a 2012 study on elite teen volleyball players. At doses of 3 grams per day, volleyball players saw increased lean muscle mass and strength during the initial phase of training.[19] There are no reported adverse effects of HMB in short-term studies of adults; few studies exist in teens, and there were none in children at the time of this writing.

Protein and Amino Acids

Athletes use protein and amino acids for a variety of reasons, but most look for effects on muscle building, increased strength, and recovery from exercise. As discussed in Chapter 2, simply consuming extra protein does not increase strength or muscle mass, but it can have a positive effect on the body's response to training. Some of the most important amino acids for sports are as follows:

Glutamine. This amino acid plays a role in immune function, and some athletes use protein supplements enriched with glutamine to improve their ability to fight infection and stay healthy.

Branched-Chain Amino Acids. These three amino acids—leucine, isoleucine, and valine—are reported to help with endurance through reducing mental fatigue, as BCAAs are involved in brain neurotransmission. There isn't enough scientific evidence at this time to support this claim.

Leucine. Ingestion of this amino acid produces a rapid increase in blood levels after exercise due to its fast absorption in the stomach and intestines. You can get leucine from the whey and casein proteins found in milk. The role of these milk proteins on exercise recovery are summarized in Chapter 2 (see page 54).

Other Amino Acids. Arginine, lysine, and ornithine stimulate the release of growth hormone and improve muscle development and strength. There is no scientific evidence that these amino acids independently increase muscle mass or strength.

Carnitine

A naturally occurring, yet essential element involved in the metabolism of fat and production of energy in the body, carnitine is naturally found in red meat, dairy products, avocado, and tempeh. It is purported to improve athletic performance, help burn fat, and produce a leaner physique. Research has found it to be ineffective at improving athletic performance, and its effectiveness as a supplement is tied to a carnitine deficiency.

Stimulants

Used as fat burners, weight-loss agents, and performance enhancers, stimulants come in a variety of forms. Some that have been banned may still be available to your athlete under different names. Three of the most common stimulants are the following:

Caffeine. Twenty-seven percent of teen athletes use caffeine for performance enhancement.[20] Caffeine increases the heart rate, raises the blood pressure, and, in adults, has been shown to increase strength, power, speed, and endurance when consumed in its pure form, such as a pill (not from coffee). Due to its addictive qualities and lack of study of its effects on children and teens, it is not recommended for them. See Chapter 4 (page 101) for more information.

Ephedra. Athletes have used this product for weight loss, appetite suppression, increased alertness, and improved performance. Side effects include high blood pressure, anxiety, tremors, headache, arrhythmias, stroke, heart attack, psychosis, and death. Banned in 2004 by the FDA, ephedra should not be used by any athlete. It is also available under the names ephedrine, ma huang, Mormon's tea, epitonin, and *Sida cordifolia*.

Bitter Orange (*Citrus Aurantium*). Milder than ephedra, this product was introduced when ephedra was banned. It is typically used for weight loss, and studies have failed to show long-term effectiveness in improving athletic performance. Chest pain, seizure, and stroke have been reported, so young athletes should avoid this product. Other names are synephrine and zhi shi.

Glycerol

Glycerol is sometimes added to beverages to help athletes hydrate better, especially in warm weather; its effect is to help the body hold water longer. When it is used as a prehydration ingredient, glycerol has been associated with stomach upset, headache, and blurred vision. Used after exercise, however, it has been shown to help correct dehydration and reduce fatigue when repeated exercise sessions occur in close succession, such as in tournament play. Use of a salt-containing sports drink is also effective at prolonging hydration. The young athlete who engages in multiple practices or competes in hot weather, like a football player, may benefit from a glycerol-based beverage, but a sports drink may be equally effective.

Vitamins and Minerals

As discussed in Chapter 3, there is no benefit to taking extra vitamin and mineral supplements beyond the Recommended Dietary Allowance (RDA), except in the case of a known nutrient deficiency. Nevertheless, many young athletes consume them. Certain micronutrients have become popular in the sports world, including the following:

Chromium. Athletes use chromium to modify their body composition—specifically, to build muscle and decrease body fat. It is typically taken in amounts much higher than the RDA. A large body of scientific evidence refutes the idea of body composition improvement and highlights potential adverse side effects, including anemia, thrombocytopenia (low amounts of white blood cells), liver impairment, renal failure, and neurologic disturbances.

Choline. Some athletes use this nutrient to improve endurance and delay fatigue, but there's a lack of scientific evidence to prove that it has those effects. Choline is found in foods such as eggs, dairy products, liver, and peanuts.

Herbal Preparations

The appeal of herbal preparations is in their supposed ability to enhance athletic performance, reduce body stress from demanding exercise, and improve immunity. Most herbal preparations are available over the counter, and most are not approved by the FDA. Many herbs can be found as ingredients in a wide variety of supplements.[21] You should be aware of them, understand their potential downsides, and investigate their inclusion in other supplements. Among the most popular of the herbs that are said to enhance athletic performance are the following:

Ginseng. Reported to improve endurance, strength, and immunity, ginseng is a central nervous system (CNS) stimulant. Research is inconclusive about its potential for enhancing athletic performance. Like caffeine, its side effects include insomnia, heart palpitations, and stomach upset. Watch out for supplements that combine ginseng and caffeine, as ginseng enhances the stimulant effects of caffeine.

Guarana. Also a CNS stimulant, guarana may be found in energy drinks along with caffeine. Guarana contains about twice the concentration of caffeine found in coffee. There is no compelling evidence that guarana enhances athletic performance, and it's not recommended for young athletes.

Echinacea. A popular herbal remedy used for the purpose of boosting the immune system and for preventing and treating the common cold, Echinacea's effectiveness in these areas is mixed. Studies in adult athletes suggest a role for Echinacea in reducing the duration of the common cold and curtailing the immune suppression that may occur with intense exercise, but more studies are needed, especially in children and teens.

Steroids

Some young athletes are tempted to use steroids, in various forms, but they are illegal without a prescription and banned for use in sports. While media coverage highlights steroid use among professional athletes, along with their negative repercussions, they aren't the only active users. Did you know that the average starting age for young athletes who use steroids is 14?[22] Rates of steroid use are reported to be 3% to 8% in boys and 0.5% to 3% in girls.[23]

Derived from testosterone, steroids are associated with building muscle mass and increasing strength and aggressiveness. Steroids may be taken orally, by injection, or applied to the skin.

The risks of steroid use are real; oral steroids are associated with liver problems, and injectable steroids pose the risk of infection, including hepatitis. In young athletes who are still growing, maturation may quicken; growth plates at the end of bones may close early, causing stunting of potential adult height; and more tendon injuries may occur.[24] Other side effects include acne, premature balding or hair loss, aggression, high blood pressure, liver damage and yellowing of the skin as a result (jaundice), and an increased risk of heart disease, blood clots, stroke, and the development of some types of cancer. Psychological effects may occur as well, such as becoming more combative or aggressive, believing things that couldn't possibly be true (delusional), and having extreme feelings of mistrust or fear (paranoia). Young athletes should not use steroids.

Ten Signs Your Athlete May Be Using Steroids

1. A recent increase in body weight, especially muscle size
2. Increase in strength
3. Acne
4. Enlarged breasts (in boys)
5. Body hair (in girls), including facial hair
6. Decreased size of breasts (in girls) and testicles (in boys)
7. Bad breath
8. Trembling
9. Mood swings, including irritability, intense anger ("roid rage"), anxiety, and depression
10. Restlessness

Prohormones

Prohormones are anabolic steroid-like substances that are reported to enhance the function of existing hormones in the body. The belief is that, upon ingestion, prohormones are converted to active hormones in the body, without incurring the drawbacks of using anabolic steroids. However, prohormones generally have the same side effects of steroids.

Dehydroepiandrosterone. Dehydroepiandrosterone (DHEA) is a precursor of testosterone and estrogen. Once a prescription drug (prior to the Dietary Supplement Health and Education Act of 1994), DHEA is now available over the counter, and the FDA does not ban its sale. DHEA has not been proven to have muscle-building effects, and is considered unsafe and ineffective. Teens sometimes use it as a substitute for steroids, and it should be regarded as a steroid. Negative side effects associated with using DHEA include irreversible gynecomastia (enlarged breast tissue) in males and unwanted hair growth in females.

Androstenedione. This steroid-like substance is found in Scotch pine tree pollen and is used as an alternative to steroids. It is said to boost testosterone levels and enhance muscle building, but research has not proven this claim. Its long-term safety is unknown, and it is banned by the FDA. It may be unknowingly packaged with other ingredients such as caffeine and stimulants. The side effects of androstenedione are similar to those of steroids.

Human Growth Hormone. Used to increase muscle mass and strength (although there is no solid scientific evidence to support this), HGH is often combined with anabolic steroids. It is often obtained illegally (without prescription) through online resources.

Weighing the Risks

The above discussion served as a primer on the most common supplements used by young athletes, as well as their performance-enhancing claims, potential risks, and where the research stands in evaluating whether they should be used or not. Now you must consider the question of what you would do if your young athlete asks to use a supplement, like David did in the case example that began the chapter. How will you respond, and how will you determine your next steps? In your quest to find information, you will want answers to these basic questions: Has the ingredient or substance been tested in young athletes? Is it safe? Is it effective? Is the supplement potentially contaminated? What are the reasons my athlete wants to use it? Will it contribute to his future use of other supplements?

Asking these questions will help you decide the right approach to take with your athlete. The good news is that athletes don't need supplements to improve performance or to get lean. Young athletes can get these results with good nutrition and exercise—knowing what to eat, what to stay away from, and when to eat, all of which I've covered earlier in this book. You always have food as a viable (reliable and safe) option to help your athlete achieve his or her performance goals.

The bad news is that young athletes often ignore their parents' and coaches' advice on the topic of supplements and take matters into their own hands. "The most dangerous supplements, such as steroids, are likely to be used by the athlete in secret, so parents and coaches need to pay attention and ask questions," warns Heather Mangieri of Nutrition CheckUp.

Investigating supplements will help you clarify your stance on supplement use and ultimately help your young athlete. Familiarity with testing and safety issues, the availability of supplements, their toxicity, the possibility of contamination, and the claims made by their manufacturers will help you assess the appropriateness of a supplement for your athlete.

Testing and Safety

When it comes to supplements, most of the testing and safety information we have comes from studies in adults. Applying what we know about adults' use of sports nutrition and supplements to growing children and teens is inappropriate and can lead to the misuse of supplements by young people. We don't really know how the body of the growing child or teenager handles or responds to supplements; hence, leading youth- and sports-oriented organizations recommend avoiding them.

Why isn't there more research on the effects of supplements on young people? Subjecting young athletes to experimental research on safety and the efficacy of supplements is considered unethical as it involves giving young people potentially dangerous doses that may interrupt their growth and cause bodily harm or worse.

Where Can I Find Reliable Information about Supplements?

There are several good resources that you can use as you gather information and make decisions about whether supplements—ranging from common compounds like protein powders to brand-new, never-heard-of-concoctions—have been tested and are certified as safe. The following companies perform screening and testing of ingredients, potency, and purity, and offer certifications of quality: NSF International (formerly the National Sanitation Foundation; www.nsf.org), United States Pharmacopeia (www.usp.org), and Consumer Lab (www.consumerlab.com). Other Internet resources that can help you assess supplements further include the Natural Medicine Comprehensive Database (www.naturaldatabase.com), and Supplement Watch (www.supplementwatch.com).

Accessibility

Young athletes have a remarkable ability to get just about anything they want in the wide world of supplements, and this should make you worry a bit. What is most concerning is the over-the-counter status of many products. Your teen can cruise through the health food aisle and pick up energy drinks, protein powders, and much more, without any restrictions. Additionally, and unfortunately, online sources offer illegal substances, such as growth hormone and steroids, and make them easy to get.[24]

Toxicity

The liver cleans toxins from the body. High levels of harmful ingredients or supplement doses may cause damage to the liver. Liver toxicity occurs in 2% to 10% of athletes using dietary supplements (energy drinks, vitamins, amino acids, and such).[25] It occurs in various forms, ranging from changes in the liver's structure (with or without symptoms) to full-blown hepatitis and even death, and thus should be a real concern for supplement users.

In addition to liver damage, anabolic steroids are associated with heart disease, reproductive problems, and premature death.[26] As mentioned earlier, athletes using steroids have been noted to be more aggressive (which some find desirable in the athletic arena), and to experience more depression and other mood disturbances than those who don't use them. Human growth hormone is also considered dangerous when it is used without a prescription. It carries a 30% risk of death even when it is prescribed and monitored by a doctor. This risk may increase when a physician is left out of the loop. Even scarier, steroids and growth hormone may be present in over-the-counter supplements as contaminants (see below). Table 7-1 identifies other supplement ingredients that can prove dangerous to the young athlete.

Finally, the effects of combining different supplement products, which many athletes attempt to do, are unknown. In one reported case study, a 17-year-old boy went to his doctor with symptoms similar to those of advanced alcoholism, including nausea, lack of appetite, a swollen liver, jaundice (yellowing of the skin), and dark urine. After an extensive medical workup that failed to discover a reason for his symptoms, the teen

Table 7-1 Supplements that Have Been Found to Be Dangerous

Supplement	Potential Danger
White willow bark	May cause bleeding and contribute to ulcers; avoid this if you cannot take aspirin
Gamma hydroxylbutyrate (GHB)	May cause seizures, coma, or death
Gamma butyrolactone (GBL)	May cause seizure, coma, or death
Rest-Eze (furanone dihydro)	May cause seizure, coma, or death
Star Caps (contains the diuretic Lasix)	May cause significant dehydration and electrolyte loss
Dieter's tea (contain senna and cascara)	May cause significant diarrhea, dehydration, and electrolyte losses
Yohimbe	May contribute to high blood pressure; toxic to kidneys
Herbs: comfrey, chaparral, germander	May be toxic to the kidneys

admitted to daily use of three different supplements over the prior 3 months: carnitine, growth hormone, and an energy drink that contained amino acids, caffeine, and creatine. He was hospitalized for treatment, and full recovery took several months.[27]

Unfortunately, many young athletes who use supplements use more than one, despite the fact that combining supplements is an extremely dangerous practice.

Contamination

High school athletes who add scoops of imported protein powder from Mexico to their sports drink may not realize that they are getting more than amino acids; the product could contain contaminants like growth hormone, trace amounts of steroids, or other ingredients that aren't identified on the label but are prohibited by doping regulations at the college and elite levels. Such additives may be included in the product due to manufacturing sloppiness or mistakes or sometimes even intentional modifications.

Up to 25% of supplements may be contaminated, according to a 2001 International Olympic Committee (IOC) study that looked at over 600 over-the-counter supplements.[28] Common contaminants include caffeine, ephedrine, and other stimulants; anabolic steroids; prohormones; and other banned substances. "There are 50,000 [supplements]. You can't tell what's in them just by studying the label," said Dr. Don Catlin, an expert on doping in sports, in a 2012 interview with ESPN.[29]

Potential contaminants pose an obvious danger to young athletes. Who wants their 12-year-old soccer player unknowingly taking steroids or their 15-year-old gymnast naively ingesting weight-loss stimulants? And taking illegal substances, knowingly or unknowingly, can potentially damage the career of the aspiring collegiate athlete or high-level competitor. At the college level, the onus is on the athlete to know what he or she is eating, as even accidental ingestion of a contaminant is subject to penalty.

The Gateway Theory

Your young athlete is still developing habits, including around supplement use. What he does now may seep into his later behavior as an athlete. Casual use of supplements in high school can evolve into a bad habit at the college level. Although there is a move to drug-test high school athletes, less than 20% of high schools across the nation do so. And those that do test are looking for alcohol, marijuana, and cocaine, not for steroids or other illegal supplements.[30]

Legal supplements may be a stepping-stone to more advanced (and dangerous) illegal supplement use. Today's choice fuels tomorrow's choices—that is essentially the premise of the Gateway Theory; early exposure to performance-enhancing supplements may open the gate to future use of supplements, perhaps illegal ones like anabolic steroids, growth hormone, or erythropoietin, which stimulates the growth of red blood cells. In a survey of over 15,000 respondents, young athletes who used legal supplements were *26 times more likely* to use anabolic steroids later on.[31]

Claims

The hook for young athletes considering supplements is the promise, delivered through advertising and marketing, of being a more accomplished athlete. Performance-enhancing supplements tout an array of claims such as the following:

- Builds muscle mass
- Improves strength
- Increases endurance
- Wards off fatigue
- Builds a healthy immune system
- Minimizes sore muscles after exercise
- Promotes quick recovery from exercise

Many of these claims are unfounded. Simply put, they add up to empty promises with little, if any, scientific evidence to back them up. But, boy, are they enticing!

When you see or hear performance-enhancing claims for supplements, be a doubting Thomas. Refuse to believe without evidence. Question the claims and—using the resources from this chapter, including the Internet sources listed on page 164—take a look at the ingredients, matching them with real evidence and information. And remember, *natural* does not mean *safe*; after all, some plants from nature are toxic when ingested.

Managing Supplements in the Young Athlete

Most adults take a conservative approach to supplements. But your young athletes may be gung-ho, ready to take on the next great miracle aid to improve their athleticism or appearance. When the fastest runner on the track team is using a "special drink" or the captain of the wrestling team downs an energy shot before hitting the mat, you better believe these actions influence the other team members. Such influences may be stronger and more powerful than your conservative, danger-avoiding approach. How will you manage these influences and help steer your athlete down the right path?

Aside from rattling off the dangers of supplements or pointing to horror stories in the news about accidental overdoses, deaths, and squelched careers related to illegal supplements (think track star Marion Jones and cyclist Lance Armstrong), there are some things you can do. But they are hard to do alone. You need a village, a policy, and awareness education to help you.

Create Your Village

The phrase "It takes a village" is a mantra worth pursuing when it comes to managing supplements in athletes. The village—a group of interested individuals whose focus is on monitoring and protecting athletes—can function as the mouth and the muscle behind the logic and the evidence. The village can consist of you, other parents, your athlete's coaching staff, the school, and your family physician. Bring these members on board to develop a cohesive approach to protecting, educating, and policing the use of supplements among the young athletes you know.

Parents are the first line of defense when a young athlete broaches the topic of supplements. You also should have your ear to the ground and remain alert for changes in case your athlete isn't forthcoming about what he or she is doing. Let your athlete know that you're aware of supplements, that you can be a resource, and that you have a well-thought-out position on them. Other team parents can be your helpers, letting you know what they are hearing about supplement use from their own athletes and other members of the team.

The coaching staff and other members of the athletic program should be aware of supplement use and should be ahead of the curve in taking charge of setting a policy on supplements for the team and intervening when supplement use is discovered. Remember the football coach in Chapter 4 who banned energy drinks when he found out his team was using them to boost their mojo before a game? He took swift action.

Keeping athletes safe is part of the job of the coach, and supplements are one of the most dangerous elements young athletes face. Schools and the athletic department can spearhead athlete education regarding supplement use early in the school year. And your family physician should be screening for supplement use at annual checkups. With this village of many vested adults and influencers addressing the issue of supplements, you have a better chance of protecting your athlete.

Establish a Policy

In my experience as a dietitian and a mother, a "just say no" policy often backfires, motivating children or teens to do the opposite of what you want them to do. However, team-wide guidelines and policies can be effective deterrents and can ease some of the pressure you're likely to feel if you're on your own as you attempt to police your own athletes. All coaches and teams should have a written policy on supplements. It should include specific guidelines for making a supplement acceptable versus unacceptable, clearly explain the team stance on the use of supplements, and lay out in no uncertain terms the actions that will be taken in the event an athlete is found to be using illegal supplements. This policy should include valid resources for athletes and their parents; should be posted in an easy-to-access forum, such as on a website; and should be reviewed at the start of each season.

Educate

Education builds awareness. Young athletes, especially teens, may not be terribly interested in statistics, but they will listen to stories of supplements gone awry and of athletes losing their careers because of supplement abuse. Accounts of women growing beards and men growing breast tissue may be enough to dissuade your athlete from using dangerous supplements. You and I know the dangers behind supplements, but you'll want to make sure your educational techniques are relevant and interesting to the young athlete; otherwise, the information may go in one ear and out the other.

The lure of supplements is real and powerful. One way to mold behavior in teens is to point them to alternative, real-food sources of the nutrients that are contained in popular supplements like protein powders, creatine, and micronutrients. Table 7-2 offers food substitutes for these common supplements. These can be easy, low-cost swaps for fancy, expensive supplements.

Accountability

One workable approach to keeping young athletes supplement-free is to ask them to sign a contract or written agreement at the beginning of the

Table 7-2 Food Swaps for Supplements

Instead of...	Try...
Creatine	Beef, poultry, and fish
Protein powders: concentrates, isolates, and hydrolysates* (whey, soy, egg, rice, pea, and others)	Milk (contains casein, whey, leucine) sources: milk, yogurt Soy sources: edamame, tofu, soymilk Eggs White or brown rice, rice milk Peas, beans Other natural protein foods such as beef, poultry, fish, nuts, and nut butter
Beta-hydroxy-beta-methylbutyrate (HMB)	Catfish, citrus fruits like orange, grapefruit
Vitamins and minerals	A variety of food sources found in Table 3-1
Stimulants	Well-balanced meals and snacks scheduled every 3–4 hours will keep your athlete energized for sport.

*Protein concentrates contain less protein and added carbs and fat; isolates are a pure form of protein, containing 90% protein; protein hydrolysates are the purest protein available and are partially digested for easier absorption.

season. Parents can do this individually, with each of their children, or coaches can draw up an agreement for the whole team.

This contract may outline specific steps an athlete must take before using a supplement, such as discussing it with the coach first. Athletes who may be taking over-the-counter supplements can keep a log of the types they are taking, as well as any prescription medications, so that potential drug interactions can be identified.

There should be discussion of the side effects of supplements, and the contract or agreement should ask the athletes to agree to inform their parents or their coach if they experience side effects like a racing heart, headache, or nausea. Have your athlete agree to discontinue supplement use should these occur. While you may not be able to prevent your athlete from trying a supplement, you can certainly set up boundaries to keep him or her safe. And, of course, you can always "say no," especially when health, safety, and legality are at issue.

Supplements are a reality of today's youth sports landscape. They can catch you off guard and cause a lot of worry, but they don't have to. Understanding the vast array of supplements available to your athlete, developing guidelines for their use, and keeping the lines of communication open are the keys to avoiding disaster.

Remember, there's no magic bullet (or pill) for enhancing performance, and especially for young athletes, there's more danger than an upside to be gained from using them. Building muscle, increasing performance and endurance, and being a top-notch young athlete comes from good nutrition and hard work. It's really as simple and as safe as that.

Notes

1. Eisenberg ME, Wall M, and Neumark-Sztainer D. "Muscle-enhancing behaviors among adolescent girls and boys." *Pediatrics.* 130 (2012): 1019–1026.
2. Ibid.
3. Goldberg C. "Full report and key findings: The 2012 Partnership Attitude Tracking Study, sponsored by MetLife Foundation." Partnership for Drug-free Kids. http://www.drugfree.org/newsroom/full-report-and-key-findings -the-2012-partnership-attitude-tracking-study-sponsored-by-metlife -foundation/.
4. Lariviere D. "Nutritional supplements flexing muscles as growth industry." *Forbes.* http://www.forbes.com/sites/davidlariviere/2013/04/18/nutritional -supplements-flexing-their-muscles-as-growth-industry/.
5. Schultz H. "Global sports nutrition industry to top 6 billion by 2018, report says." Food Navigator-USA.com. http://www.foodnavigator-usa.com/ Markets/Global-sports-nutrition-market-to-top-6-billion-by-2018-report -says.
6. Evans MW, Ndetan H, Perko M, Williams R, and Walker C. "Dietary supplement use by children and adolescents in the United States to enhance sport performance: results of the National Health Interview Survey." *J Primary Prevent.* 33 (2012): 3–12.
7. Lattavo A, Kopperud A, and Rogers PD. "Creatine and other supplements." *Pediatr Clin N Am.* 54 (2007): 735–760.
8. Ibid, p. 736.
9. Ibid, p. 737.
10. Rosenbloom CA and Coleman EJ, eds. *Sports Nutrition: A Practice Manual for Professionals,* 5th ed. Chicago: Academy of Nutrition and Dietetics, 2012.
11. McDowell J. "Supplement use by young athletes." *J Sports Sci Med.* 6 (2007): 337–342.

12. Dodge TL and Jaccard JJ. "The effect of high school sports participation on the use of performance-enhancing substances in young adulthood." *J Adolesc Health.* 39 (2006): 367–373.

13. Dunn M, Eddy JM, Wang MQ, Nagy S, Perko MA, and Bartee T. "The influence of significant others on attitudes, subjective norms and intentions regarding dietary supplement use among adolescent athletes." *Adolescence.* 36 (2001): 583–591.

14. Calfee R and Fadale P. "Popular ergogenic drugs and supplements in young athletes." *Pediatrics.* 117 (2006): 577–589.

15. Metzl JD, Small E, Levine SR, and Gershel JC. "Creatine use among young athletes." *Pediatrics.* 108 (2001): 421–425.

16. Cooper R, Naclerio F, Allgrove J, and Jimenez A. "Creatine supplementation with specific view to exercise/sports performance: an update." *J Int Society Sports Nutr.* 9 (2012): 33.

17. Wilson JM, Fitschen PJ, Campbell B, Wilson GJ, Zanchi N, Taylor L, Wilborn C, Kalman DS, Stout JR, Hoffman JR, Ziegenfuss TN, Lopez HL, Kreider RB, Smith-Ryan AE, and Antonio J. "International Society of Sports Nutrition Position Stand: beta-hydroxy-beta-methylbutyrate (HMB)." *J Int Soc Sports Nutr.* 10 (2013): 6.

18. Lattavo, op. cit, p. 747.

19. Portal S, Zadik Z, Rabinowitz J, Pilz-Burstein R, Adler-Portal D, Meckel Y, Cooper DM, Eliakim A, and Nemet D. "The effect of HMB supplementation on body composition, fitness, hormonal and inflammatory mediators in elite adolescent volleyball players: a prospective, randomized, double-blind, placebo-controlled study." *Eur J Appl Physiol.* 111 (2011): 2261–2269.

20. Lattavo, op. cit, p. 749.

21. Senchina D. "Athletics and herbal supplements. Do current products enhance athletes' health and performance?" *American Scientist.* http://www.americanscientist.org/issues/feature/athletics-and-herbal-supplements/1.

22. Lorang M, Callahan B, Cummins KM, Achar S, and Brown SA. "Anabolic androgenic steroid use in teens: prevalence, demographics, and perceptions of effects." *J Child Adolesc Substance Abuse.* 20 (2011): 358–369.

23. Greydanus DE and Patel DR. "Sports doping in the adolescent: the Faustian conundrum or hors de combat." Pediatr Clin N Am. 57 (2010): 729–750.

24. Shipley A. "Study finds steroids in supplements easily purchased online." *Washington Post.* http://www.washingtonpost.com/wp-dyn/content/article/2011/01/18/AR2011011805861.html.

25. Stickel F, Kessebohm K, Weimann R, and Seitz H. "Review of liver injury associated with dietary supplements." *Liver Int.* 31 (2011): 595–605.

26. Ibid. 22, p. 735.

27. Avelar-Escobar G, Mendez-Navarro J, Ortiz-Olvera NX, Castellanos G, Ramos, R, Gallardo-Cabrera VE, Vargas-Aleman J, Diaz de Leon O, Rodriguez EV, and Dehesa-Violante M. "Hepatotoxicity associated with dietary energy supplements: use and abuse by young athletes." *Ann Hepatol.* 11 (2012): 564–569.

28. Schanzer W. "Analysis of non-hormonal nutritional supplements for anabolic-androgenic steroids: an international study." Olympic.org Official website of the Olympic Movement. http://www.olympic.org/Documents/Reports/EN/en_report_324.pdf.

29. Newton D. "Supplement contamination common." ESPN Nascar. http://espn.go.com/racing/nascar/cup/story/_/id/8179792/nascar-aj-allmendinger-easily-taken-contaminated-supplement.

30. Centers for Disease Control and Prevention. School Health Policies and Practices Study (SHPPS). "SHPPS 2006 school level data files." http://www.cdc.gov/healthyYouth/shpps/2006/data/school.htm.

31. Ibid. 7, pg. 755.

PART III

Clearing the Hurdles

CHAPTER 8

Getting Off the Bench— Healing the Body with Food

Let food be thy medicine and medicine be thy food.
—Hippocrates

Andrew was a stellar high school hockey player. As a varsity starter, he got a lot of playing time. When he took a hard hit to his head, his doctor and coach benched him. "What do I do now?" asked Andrew. "I'm on bed rest for a week or two and won't be back on the ice for at least a month."

What Andrew had to do was change his nutrition plan. Bed rest meant no exercise, which translated to lower calorie needs and less eating. That's not easy for a young guy who's used to several hours of hard exercise several days a week. Andrew's norm was to eat whatever, whenever, and however much he wanted, so cutting back was a challenge. Nutrition didn't play a big role in the management of his concussion per se, but it was important nevertheless. Adjusting Andrew's daily diet could prevent unwanted weight gain and help him stay ready for the action when he recovered.

Many health obstacles can cause problems for young athletes, including injury, bone breaks, and weight challenges. Nutrition—the cornerstone of health and wellness for all people—is a key ingredient in maintaining health, preventing medical problems, and helping athletes recover from illness or injury.

This chapter explores some of the most common effects of poor nutrition for young athletes, including weight problems, eating disorders, overuse injury and bone fractures, and growth delay. It provides nutrition recommendations for dealing with these issues and will help you understand when more help is needed. I'll also discuss chronic medical conditions such as diabetes, celiac disease, and food allergies, and showcase the latest strategies for athletes managing these challenges.

Common Hurdles Set Up by Inadequate Nutrition

Suzie carried extra weight that she and her coach wished she would lose. Martin, a cross-country athlete, was too thin, and wanted to gain some weight. Gretchen had an eating disorder, yet still maintained a rigorous dance schedule and showed up for competitions. From carrying too much or too little weight to dealing with an eating disorder or the side effects of poor nutrition, young athletes face a number of obstacles that are related to nutrition. You can prevent many of these hiccups, but some will happen despite your best efforts. But good nutrition, along with adequate sleep and good hygiene, can minimize, maybe even prevent, and even heal many issues that may sideline your athlete. Let's look at the most common nutrition-related obstacles, such as overweight and obesity, underweight, eating disorders, and the female athlete triad, and explore some of the options available to help allay their effects.

Overweight and Obesity

National studies demonstrate that more than a quarter of youth sport participants (26% of boys and 27% of girls) are overweight, and nearly half (48%) of young people who are obese say they participate in sports.[1] Many children start to play a sport for the side benefit of managing their weight, yet there is no guarantee athletes will shed pounds this way, or even avoid obesity.[2] In fact, being overweight carries a higher risk: it doubles the likelihood of sports injuries, mostly involving the knee.[3,4] Despite these facts, physical activity is *always* part of the plan for an overweight child or teen, as research shows a combination of physical activity and balanced, healthy eating helps kids and teens normalize their weight and improve their health.

Weight Status Versus Body Fatness in Young Athletes

As discussed in Chapter 1, body mass index (BMI)—a measure of total body weight related to height—is often displayed on a BMI growth chart for children and teens at physicians' offices, or you can view one at www.cdc.gov/growthcharts/. "Overweight" means the BMI falls between the 85th and 95th percentiles, and "obese" reflects a BMI falling above the 95th percentile.

Often the BMI is interpreted as a measure of fatness, but this is a tricky read for young athletes because the BMI fails to tell us about body composition—lean tissue (muscle and bone) versus fat. People often associate body composition, especially leanness, with better performance outcomes, and, truth be told, studies do support this association.

Athletes with normal BMIs can have bodies with too much fat or too little fat. In a 2012 study of female high school athletes, researchers found that subjects with normal BMI had both low body fat levels (2% had less than 12% body fat) and high body fat levels (6.7% had more than 33% body fat). Athletes who had low body fat levels reported stress fractures and use of weight-control agents, such as laxatives; 57% of these athletes were diagnosed with a clinical eating disorder or low bone density. The athletes with high body fat reported engaging in unhealthy weight-loss measures and disorders related to the female athlete triad. Forty-seven percent were diagnosed with an eating disorder.[5]

The BMI is only one indicator of your athlete's weight status. There will always be bigger, more muscular athletes who have low body fat, thin athletes with high body fat, and everything in between. The goal is to be at a healthy weight with a healthy body fat level that contributes to athletic abilities. Healthy body fat levels are as follows: for preteen boys, 12% to 20%; for preteen girls, 14% to 28%; for teenage boys, 10% to 22%; and for teenage girls, 20% to 32%. Teenage boys should stay above a minimum body fat level of 7% and teenage girls should stay above 14%.[6]

While the BMI is the easiest and most accessible means to assess body fatness, it isn't always ideal for the serious or elite young athlete. Other means of assessing body composition include waist circumference measurements (useful for measuring abdominal fat), waist-to-hip ratio (also measures abdominal obesity), skinfold thickness (a caliper measures the thickness of a pinch of skin at various areas of the body, such as the shoulder blade, trunk, upper thigh, and back of the upper arm), and bioelectrical impedance (BIA; an imperceptible, safe, and small electrical current is sent through the body; it passes slowly through fat tissue and quickly through muscle and bone; equations are used to calculate body fatness and lean tissue). Air-displacement plethysmography (one commercial machine is called BodPod) involves sitting in a small chamber wearing a bathing suit; the machine estimates body volume based on air pressure differences within the chamber. These methods can be done in a clinic or community setting, and are done in research settings too. More sophisticated methods such as magnetic resonance imaging (MRI) and dual-energy X-ray absorptiometry (DEXA) are typically done in research settings.

Exercise alone may not be enough to produce weight loss. "My son started playing soccer this year for two reasons: to have fun and to shed some pounds," said Patrick, father of 9-year-old Luke. "He's definitely having fun, but I don't see the weight coming off." When we talked about what Luke was eating, it was clear that getting a handle on his food and eating habits would be the key to helping him. Like many young athletes, Luke was eating too many snacks and sweets. Cleaning up this part of his diet would allow exercise to tip the energy balance to a better place so that he could experience a gradual weight loss over time.

The top two problematic food categories for young athletes are fast food and sugary sweet drinks such as soda, juice, and sports drinks.[7] Abundant in empty calories (especially soda) or overconsumed, these foods are major contributors to weight gain. The inclusion of sports drinks with meals and snacks has been identified as problematic, according to the Committee on Nutrition and the Council on Sports Medicine and Fitness.[8] The committee recommends that children *avoid* sports drinks during meals, snacks, and as a replacement for low-fat milk or water because they increase the risk for overweight or obesity. If you do nothing else, encourage your children to say good-bye to fast food and sugary drinks.

If you embark on a plan for weight change for your young athlete, keep these facts in mind:

- Young athletes are still growing, and you want to safeguard that process.
- Dramatically changing the diet can have negative effects on stamina.
- Significant weight change during a sport season can have an undesirable impact on performance.

Ideally, you'll want a nutrition plan that offers an adequate supply of nutrients and calories so that your athlete keeps growing normally and his or her athletic performance is unharmed.

Reducing fat and the refined sugar found in sweets and sugary beverages is the safest and easiest way to approach dietary changes, as often these are the culprits when it comes to extra calories.[9] As discussed in Chapter 2, fat is the nutrient to cut back on when a young athlete wants to lose weight, as a diet lower in fat permits calorie reduction without compromising carbohydrate and protein intake. Shoot for a diet that is high in whole fruits and vegetables and whole grains, and that includes low-fat dairy, beans, and lean meats. For a refresher on healthy eating, see Chapters 5 and 6. Table 8-1 details the do's and don'ts of managing the young athlete's weight.

Remember, managing weight is a two-pronged approach: exercise and balanced nutrition. Exercise won't correct an unhealthy diet. You'll need to pay attention to both aspects to help your athlete achieve and maintain a healthy weight.

Underweight

Some athletes struggle with being underweight. Elizabeth's son Bart was tall and thin. As a basketball player, his height was advantageous, but his low weight concerned her. "He's a bit picky and doesn't seem to eat enough, especially during basketball season," she said. "He wants to gain

Table 8-1 The Do's and Don'ts of Weight Management in the Young Athlete

Do	Reason
Eat breakfast	Helps to replenish glycogen after an overnight fast; provides fuel for exercise; regulates food intake through the day
Spread food intake throughout the day	Helps to manage hunger; ensures optimal nutrients are available throughout the day
Eat after exercise	Helps with exercise recovery; may stave off excess hunger
Get rid of sugary drinks	Cuts down on empty calories; may reduce cravings for sweets
Avoid fad diets	Quick fix diets don't work; may cause weight gain in the long run, and dehydration in the short-term
Include low-fat, high-quality protein	Provides feeling of fullness; lower in calories than higher fat versions
Include fiber	Contributes to fullness
Eat nutrient-rich foods	Whole grains, fruit, and vegetables offer a lot of nutrition without a lot of calories
Don't	**Reason**
Drink sugary drinks and alcohol	Adds extra calories without increasing fullness, improving nutrient intake or curtailing food consumption
Slash calories (severely)	Combined with endurance and strength training, severe calorie reduction may diminish weight loss, as body tries to conserve energy; causes excess hunger and extreme stress to the athlete body
Fast, or not eat	Under-fuels body and may cause extreme hunger and overeating; may contribute to muscle loss
Eliminate food groups or major nutrients (carbs) from the diet	May cause nutrient deficits over time; eliminating carbs may negatively impact performance
Use extreme weight control behaviors (diuretics, laxatives, vomiting, etc.)	May become habitual and lead to an eating disorder; electrolyte abnormalities; nutrient deficiencies; dehydration; negatively affects performance
Restrict fluids	May cause dehydration and potential electrolyte losses; weight loss is temporary

weight, and I think it will help him be stronger and have more stamina."
Whether your young athletes are genetically predisposed to thinness, like
Bart is, or are underweight from a combination of poor eating and exercise, a little bit of weight gain will help them feel stronger and sleep better, and it may help their athletic performance.

Adding a nightly snack to the daily routine and "padding" calories into
foods are two ways to increase calories in the diet. A homemade or commercial shake or a hearty snack before bedtime can offer the extra calories
your athlete needs. Padding sandwiches with high-calorie spreads—
mayonnaise, butter, or avocado, another slice of cheese, or more nut
butter—can build extra calories into an athlete's diet without asking him
or her to eat huge portions. Getting your athlete to gain weight takes
planning and consistency. Table 8-2 lists more ideas to help your athlete
add pounds.

Table 8-2 Eight Ways to Help Young Athletes Gain Weight

Start providing a bedtime snack	Any combination of protein, carbohydrate, and fat will add nutritious calories to your athletes diet. Check Chapter 6 for ideas.
Pad foods with extra calories	Extra butter, olive oil, peanut butter, cheese, and other high-calorie condiments or add-ons can boost total calories.
Choose high-calorie foods	Nix the reduced or low fat items. Full fat dairy products such as milk, yogurt, cream, sour cream, and cheese will be higher in calories.
Add spreads that have calories	Mayonnaise, butter, cream cheese, nut butter, and avocado can add additional calories to a sandwich.
Double-dress the grains	Toss pasta or other grains in olive oil before layering on other sauces such as Alfredo or marinara sauce.
Add a protein punch	Toss in an extra egg in baked goods like cookies, pancakes, cakes, and other desserts. Powdered milk can be added to milk-based drinks and baked goods.
Serve larger portions	Eating more food volume will give your athlete more calories. Inch up on portion sizes, especially with high-calorie foods.
Don't dilute	Make 100% juice, other ready-to-mix beverages, and soups with a little less water to increase the calorie content.

Eating Disorders

Kelly was a track-and-field athlete whose troubles began during her junior year, when she decided she wanted to lose weight. To achieve her goal, she skipped meals and dieted during the school week and ran extra miles after practice. On the weekends, she binged on cookies, chips, frozen entrées, bread, and alcohol, and compensated for "ruining my good diet" by purging (vomiting). Despite her extreme weight-loss efforts, her weight remained unchanged, which unfortunately fueled her unhealthy behaviors. Eventually, she did lose a little bit of weight, but she developed some serious medical complications along the way. She was diagnosed with an eating disorder, and her running career and social life were put on hold while she received treatment.

Some athletes like Kelly strive for a lean physique using food restriction, unhealthy weight-control measures, and over-exercising, but in doing so they run the risk of something more serious—an eating disorder. Eating disorders can start as early as age 9 in both sexes. They generally begin with *disordered eating*, which means the athlete imposes seemingly harmless restrictions on his or her eating in an effort to control or lose body weight.[10]

Signs of disordered eating include avoiding certain types of food; restricting amounts of food, which can result in eating less than is needed for growth and training; bingeing; purging; and using weight-loss crutches such as laxatives, diuretics, stimulants, and appetite suppressants. Since disordered eating is a precursor to a full-scale eating disorder, you'll want to keep your eye on any unhealthy or unproductive eating behaviors that you see developing in your child or teen. While it doesn't mean your athlete *has* an eating disorder, disordered eating that persists can morph into something much more serious.

Athletes, both male and female, who participate in sports with an aesthetic component, such as gymnastics, ice skating, and dancing; in weight-class sports such as judo and rowing; in gym sports such as aerobics; in endurance sports such as swimming; or in low-weight performance sports such as long-distance running appear to be at a higher risk for using unhealthy ways to control or reduce their body weight.[11] In weight-class and aesthetic sports, about 62% of girls have disordered eating, and 33% of boys are affected by eating disorders.[12]

Risk factors that can make a young athlete vulnerable to an eating disorder include the following:

*   An emphasis on appearance, weight requirements, or muscularity: at risk are athletes who participate in gymnastics, diving, bodybuilding, and wrestling.
*   An individual sport rather than a team sport: at risk are athletes who participate in gymnastics, running, figure skating, dance, and diving.
*   Endurance sports: at risk are athletes who participate in track and field, running, and swimming.
*   A "lean athlete" mentality, that is, a belief that a lower body weight will result in better performance: at risk are all athletes.
*   Elite status or specialization from a young age.
*   Low self-esteem, a family history of an eating disorder, family and cultural pressure, trauma.

Female athletes, particularly, experience additional factors, such as societal pressure to be thin, performance anxiety, and negative self-perception of their athletic performance, which make them more susceptible to disordered eating and potentially an eating disorder.

A Word on Body Image

Self-esteem and body image develop during childhood and adolescence. Playing sports has been linked to a positive body image and higher self-esteem, but some athletes struggle with poor body image. Being concerned about body weight, shape, and size can influence eating behaviors—particularly in teens, whose bodies undergo rapid changes and growth spurts—and this concern may lead to unhealthy weight-control practices, such as unnecessary dieting, disordered eating, or an eating disorder. Be aware that the pressure to be thin, athletic, and perfect in every way may chip away at your athlete's body image and self-esteem. Protect your athlete by de-emphasizing thinness and appearance, focusing instead on the other benefits of exercise, such as feeling healthy, fit, and strong, stress relief and mood enhancement, and better sleep.

Anorexia nervosa, bulimia nervosa, and binge-eating disorder are official eating disorders, with specific diagnostic criteria that are outlined below. Eating-disorder characteristics that don't fall into a well-defined category for diagnosis are identified as eating disorder not otherwise specified (EDNOS). Below are the typical traits you will find for each:

Anorexia Nervosa. Characterized by deliberate self-starvation, a refusal to keep body weight at a minimally healthy level, an intense fear of gaining weight, a distorted body image, and, in girls, missing periods. Anorexia can be restrictive in nature, or it can involve binge eating and purging. Sufferers appear extremely thin and may have electrolyte and hormonal disruptions, irregular heartbeat, low blood counts, and anemia.

Bulimia Nervosa. This disorder is characterized by recurring binge eating (eating large volumes of food in a short period) followed by vomiting or another form of purging (laxatives, diuretics, fasting, or excessive exercise). Sufferers may be underweight, overweight, or normal weight; may use athletic training to mask purging; and may suffer from stomach complications, such as constipation or diarrhea, tears in the esophagus from vomiting, or dental cavities.

Binge Eating Disorder. This is recurrent binge eating without purging. The excessive intake of calories from overeating causes weight gain.

Eating Disorder Not Otherwise Specified (EDNOS). This term describes a variety of eating disorder symptoms. However, in total, these symptoms do not meet the exact criteria for either anorexia or bulimia. For example, a girl could have all the criteria for anorexia but still have her period. The following are common terms and descriptions of eating disorders that fall into the category of EDNOS:

Anorexia athletica: A term used for athletes who have eating disorder symptoms and exercise excessively but do not fall within the criteria for anorexia or bulimia.

Orthorexia nervosa: Individuals who are obsessive and extreme about eating "healthy" food.

Diabulimia: A condition whereby diabetics manipulate their insulin for the purpose of weight loss.

Drunkorexia: Characterized by self-starvation, or bingeing and purging, while abusing alcohol.

Signs of an Eating Disorder in Young Athletes

It can be hard to recognize an eating disorder in your athlete early on, partly due to the expectation and assumption that an athlete should be lean and trim, and to the fact that some signs, such as an insistence on eating only healthy foods, may seem desirable or the behaviors subtle. Be on the lookout for these common signs:

- Underweight or overweight; also normal weight (see below)
- Lack of concentration, energy, coordination, and speed
- Fatigue and increased perception of exertion
- Longer recovery time required between events
- Frequent injury
- Low blood pressure and slowed heart rate
- Low body temperature, noted by cold hands and feet
- Light-headedness and dizziness
- Perfectionism
- Impatient, cranky (more than usual)
- Prefers to be alone
- Dislikes time off from exercise; refuses tapering
- Avoids drinking water and other beverages
- Preoccupation with one's food and with other people's food
- Odd eating behaviors, food preferences, and food combinations
- Overconcern with body appearance
- Participates in additional training
- Fellow teammates concerned

One dangerous myth is that athletes with eating disorders are underweight and skinny. However, in one study, as many as 47.6% of normal-weight athletes were diagnosed with a present or past eating disorder, either bulimia nervosa or EDNOS.[13] Don't let the outer appearance of an athlete fool you into missing a serious problem. Even previously overweight individuals who have lost weight and are currently at a "normal" weight may have an eating disorder, particularly if other qualifying eating behaviors, weight-loss tactics, and physical signs (such as lack of menstruation) are present.

Female Athlete Triad

Sarah, a 15-year-old runner, told her mother that she hadn't had her period for a while. "She's been very careful about what she eats, working with her coach to cut down her body fat," reported her mom. "But I think it's gone too far. I'm upset about the no-period thing. I know that's not healthy."

Missing periods—erratically or consistently—is not normal or healthy. Menstruation is a core function in the health of females, whether or not they are athletic. Sarah needed a medical evaluation to uncover the reasons for her amenorrhea (absence of a menstrual cycle) and treatment to address them—pronto.

According to the National Eating Disorders Association (NEDA), about 66% of female athletes are not having their menstrual cycles.[14] The combination of disordered eating, lack of regular menstruation, and low bone mass is called the female athlete triad. The triad can range from a mild condition in which an athlete avoids certain foods and carefully controls her calorie intake, has irregular periods, and has experienced a stress fracture, to a more extreme case in which the athlete has anorexia, has not had a period for a long time, and has developed osteoporosis.

Disordered eating may lead to weight loss, body fat loss, and menstrual dysfunction. Missed periods occur due to low energy availability, either from inadequate eating or too much exercise. The result is a low estrogen level, which is a key ingredient for bone formation and the maintenance of bone health. A lack of menstruation should be evaluated within 3 months of when it starts; restoring monthly periods is the goal of treatment.[15]

Low bone mass is concerning, especially for girls. Bone formation peaks during the teenage years; up to 90% of girls' bones should be formed by age 18, with the remaining bone developing throughout early adulthood. It's hard to know if your athlete has low bone density without doing a dual-energy X-ray absorptiometry (DEXA) scan, but stress fractures are a hint that a girl may have low bone density. Assessing bone density, particularly if your athlete has erratic or no menstrual periods, can help prevent future osteoporosis.

Treatment for the triad is straightforward and simple, though often not easy for young athletes. It involves revising the eating plan to meet energy needs and calcium and vitamin D requirements. If the triad includes the disordered eating component, getting enough food can be a challenge. If exercise is contributing to a negative energy balance, backing off from physical activity may help restore menstruation by placing the athlete in a positive energy balance. Again, decreasing exercise may be tough for the serious athlete.

You want to be highly aware of, and suspicious of, disordered eating and eating disorders in any serious, elite athlete, particularly in sports that favor a low body weight or those that include an emphasis on physical appearance. Recognizing the early signs is the first step to curtailing these unhealthy behaviors and getting your athlete on the right track.

Treatment

Eating disorders, disordered eating, and the female athlete triad are serious conditions. Often they are too complicated for a parent or coach to handle alone. If you suspect your young athlete has an eating disorder or are concerned about disordered eating or the female athlete triad, get a medical evaluation. A physician, a registered dietitian/nutritionist, a therapist, or the combination of these professionals can be very helpful to your athlete as he or she overcomes these challenges.

Healthy eating patterns, nutritious food, a positive perspective on body image, and a good balance between exercise, rest, and play should be the foundation of any athlete's healthy life. Be vigilant and aware of these complications so you can help your young athlete keep playing and stay healthy.

Injuries and the Role of Nutrition

Young athletes aren't immune to the toll that exercise and activity can take on the growing body. Two million high school athletes are injured annually, representing 500,000 doctor visits and 30,000 hospitalizations, and over 3.5 million children under age 14 seek medical treatment for sports-related injuries every year.[16] While the potential for injury goes along with being an athlete, there are a few things you should know, and can do, to alleviate the negative impact on your athlete's ability to play. Let's take a look at how nutrition plays a role in contributing to, and healing, overuse injury and bone fractures.

Overuse Injury

According to a 2007 report in the journal *Pediatrics*, one of the most common challenges for the young athlete is overuse injury, defined as an injury to a bone, ligament, or tendon due to repetitive stress without sufficient time to heal.[17] Examples of overuse injury are stress fractures, tendonitis, and ligament tears.

As sports participation has grown in popularity, so has the incidence of overuse injury. Up to 50% of all injuries in young athletes are related to overuse. Young athletes with prior injury who are in their adolescent growth spurt and girls who have menstrual irregularities are at risk for overuse, as are those athletes who have a high training load, play a year-round sport, and have limited free play or other sport/recreational activities.

Young athletes, whose bones, ligaments, and tendons are developing and thus are susceptible to damage, are by nature prone to overuse injuries. Their growing cartilage, growth plates, and apophyses (the sites where muscle attaches to bone, such as the heel, elbow, and knee) are vulnerable to stress and are often injured. Some examples: young baseball pitchers who damage their elbow due to repetition combined with improper throwing mechanics; gymnasts who repeatedly hyperextend and develop a stress fracture of their spine (called spondylolysis); and swimmers who develop shoulder tendinitis that goes unrecognized because their symptoms—fatigue, poor performance, and vague pain—have been misinterpreted. Also, young athletes may not recognize or acknowledge the signs of injury.

How Much Is Too Much Exercise?

The American Academy of Pediatrics (AAP) recommends the following limitations for youth sports training in order to prevent overuse injury[18]:

- No more than one sporting activity, 5 days per week
- At least 1 day off each week from any organized activity
- At least 2 to 3 months off per year

High levels of training and competition place children and teens at risk for overuse injury. Year-round participation in one sport, called sports specialization, can involve repetition and infrequent breaks from training; without alternative activities, it is a setup for overuse injury. Young athletes who participate in a variety of sporting activities have fewer injuries and are motivated to play sports longer than those who specialize before puberty.[19] However, multisport athletes can also succumb to overuse injury, especially if they play sports that use similar movements and body parts, such as swimming and baseball.

Bone Fractures

Stress fractures, a type of overuse injury, are reported at a much higher rate today than ever before, an increased incidence that correlates with the popularity of youth sports.[20] The most common stress fractures in young athletes occur in the spine (spondylolysis), shinbones, thighs, toes, and feet.[21] Bone fractures in youth tend to occur because of training errors, defects in biomechanics, and dietary deficiencies; in girls, they are associated with loss of menstrual function. Athletes who participate in sports that encourage restrictive eating patterns—such as cross-country running, other track and field events, rowing, and gymnastics—may see greater incidence of stress fractures in girls with and without the female athlete triad (see page 188).[22]

A 2010 review study in high school athletes looked at the role of calcium and vitamin D in preventing stress fractures and showed that calcium intakes of 1,500 mg and 800 International Units (IU) of vitamin D daily reduced the incidence of stress fractures.[23] Another study identified vitamin D as the pivotal nutrient in preventing stress fractures among high school female athletes, although more research is needed in this area.[24] Unfortunately, teens eat far less than what is recommended for calcium and vitamin D, according to the Dietary Guidelines for Americans (DGA).[25]

Good nutrition helps prevent overuse and encourages healing. If your athlete is benched, a well-rounded, nutritious diet can help the healing process; both macronutrients (especially protein) and micronutrients (vitamins and minerals) play a supportive role in an athlete's recovery. A healthy diet, particularly one adequate in calcium and vitamin D, may help your athlete heal faster, and prevent stress fractures in the first place.

And remember that when athletes rest, their calorie needs dip to non-training levels. Athletes who are healing fall into the sedentary to moderately active category for energy needs (see Table 1-1).

Chronic Medical Challenges

Some young athletes may be dealing with lifelong health conditions such as diabetes, celiac disease, or food allergies. These medical conditions pose special challenges for growth, development, and overall health, not to mention athletic success. Managing any of these conditions makes playing a sport more challenging. However, if these young athletes keep nutrition in mind, they can be just as competitive as their peers. Let's look at the nutrition considerations for these challenges.

Diabetes

According to the American Diabetes Association, 29 million Americans had diabetes in 2012, of whom 208,000 (0.7%) were under the age of 20.[26] Diabetes, especially type 1, poses added considerations for the young athlete, particularly for the prevention of hypoglycemia (low blood sugar) during exercise.

Carly was diagnosed with type 1 diabetes at age 10. As a competitive dancer, she trains for about 14 hours each week, and more on weekends. Managing her diabetes takes center stage. "It's a constant juggling act," says her mom, Heather. "She's not like other kids—she can't really delay or skip a meal based on her performance time, so we have to make adjustments to her eating, and sometimes her insulin."

Type 1 diabetes is typically diagnosed in childhood or young adulthood. The pancreas does not produce insulin, the hormone responsible for converting sugar, starches, and other food into energy for daily living and exercise; as a result, diabetics need external insulin, delivered by injections or an insulin pump, to keep their blood sugar levels within a normal range (not too high and not too low).

While there are long-term complications of high blood sugar in the athlete with diabetes (heart disease, and nerve and kidney damage, to name a few), an imminent concern is a condition called diabetic ketoacidosis, where the blood sugar runs too high due to the body's not having enough available insulin. Diabetic ketoacidosis can cause a build up of ketones in the bloodstream, and if untreated can lead to diabetic coma, and become life threatening. The dangers of a low blood sugar are concerning for the young athlete as well (see below). For these reasons, athletes must measure their blood sugar levels frequently and adjust their insulin and/or food intake to keep their blood sugar levels stabilized.

The trick is that insulin and glucose from food must be in balance for blood sugar levels to be in a normal range. Diabetics must plan their food intake to provide a steady, even distribution of carbohydrates throughout the day to closely match the insulin that is delivered.

Exercise makes the body more efficient at using insulin and transporting glucose into the cells. However, the body's response to exercise varies based on the type of exercise. Short-duration bouts of anaerobic exercise (e.g., weight lifting) may set the stage for high blood sugar, or hyperglycemia, while aerobic exercise (e.g., soccer, running) may result in low blood sugar, called hypoglycemia.

Generally, hypoglycemia is the more common concern for athletes. Because exercise can cause greater sensitivity to insulin, hypoglycemia may occur during, shortly after, or even up to 24 hours after exercise.[27] Experts agree that most physical activity lasting longer than 30 minutes requires some adjustment in food or insulin delivery.[28] Furthermore, diabetic athletes may need up to 0.7 gram of carbohydrate per pound per hour during strenuous exercise.[29]

Athletic performance may also be compromised with poor blood sugar control. In well-controlled diabetic athletes, performance is similar to that in nondiabetic athletes; however, in poorly controlled athletes, early fatigue and poor cognitive function affect athletic performance.[30] And an athlete's risk of injury is higher with hypoglycemia. Sports that involve quick movements increase the risk for collision, and slow cognitive function can contribute to poor decision making, particularly in sports such as soccer and hockey.

In order to prevent low blood sugar, young athletes need to frequently monitor their blood sugar levels, what and when they eat, and the duration and intensity of their exercise, adjusting their insulin and food intake as needed.

Tips for Preventing Hypoglycemia in the Young Athlete with Diabetes

- Do not let your young athlete go more than 3 or 4 hours without eating a meal or a snack.
- Check his or her blood sugar before, during, and after exercise.
- Adjust the insulin dose before exercise according to the duration and intensity of exercise, as per medical guidelines.
- Be sure that your athlete increases the length and intensity of activity progressively.
- Keep a training record that details the intensity and duration of exercise and its impact on blood sugar. This will give your athlete insight into his or her body's response to exercise.
- Blood sugar should be 100 mg/dL before exercise, or a minimum level agreed upon with your health care provider. If it's lower than desired, then encourage your athlete to eat some carbs (about 15 grams).
- Be sure that your athlete always carries something to eat or drink in order to treat hypoglycemia that occurs during practice or a competition.

"Unfortunately, Carly has experienced lows during competition—always at the most inopportune time, just before she is set to go on stage," says Heather. Athletes who experience episodes of low blood sugar, like Carly, must be prepared to treat them. Fast-acting carbs (simple carbs)—glucose tablets, hard candies, cake icing, glucose gels, fruit juice, soft drinks—work well. Glucose tabs offer a controlled dosage of 4 or 5 grams of carbs. Athletes can use the "rule of 15," taking three or four glucose tabs (equivalent to 12 to 20 grams of carbs) and retesting their blood sugar 15 minutes later. They then repeat this process, as needed, to get blood sugars into target range. This systematic approach prevents an overshoot of carbs and subsequent high blood sugar.

Other complications of diabetes affecting athletes include high blood pressure, which can contribute to headaches, and eye problems, which can blur or obstruct vision. Nutritionally, young athletes with diabetes should guard against stress fractures with a diet rich in calcium and vitamin D, as low bone mineral content is associated with diabetes. Diabetes can also cause the production of free radicals (cell-damaging elements) in the body, which may damage the retina in the eye and cause other nerve problems, so make sure to include antioxidant-rich foods containing vitamin C, vitamin E, and selenium in your athlete's diet (for food sources of these micronutrients, see Chapter 3). Finally, athletes should avoid loading up on protein supplements, as they can produce excess calories, which may raise blood sugar levels.

The athlete with diabetes should eat like a nondiabetic athlete (one, of course, who follows a sound nutritional program), with a couple of caveats. In addition to regular meals and snacks; a balanced blend of carbs, protein, and fat; and regular timing, you'll want to pay close attention to distributing carbs evenly throughout the day in your athlete's diet. Time meals and snacks to occur anywhere between 1 and 4 hours prior to exercise, depending on your athlete's digestion, tolerance of eating pre-exercise food, and blood sugar levels. Preloading with a carb-based snack depends on the current blood sugar level and the exercise plan. If blood sugar is greater than 150 mg/dL before exercise, athletes with diabetes probably don't need to top off with a carb-based snack, but they may need some carbs during exercise, depending on how strenuously and how long they plan to exercise.

During exercise, athletes may need to consume 0.5 to 0.7 grams of carbohydrate per pound, depending on the insulin dose and peak insulin activity.[31] This can be done with a carbohydrate-based beverage such as a sports drink, or with food. Tables 2-1 and 2-2 in Chapter 2 list the carb loads of selected foods. If exercise lasts longer than 60 minutes, make sure your athlete has a high-carb recovery snack at hand so he or she can take advantage of heightened insulin sensitivity, as this allows rapid glycogen replenishment and prevents post-exercise low blood sugar.[32] Also, remind your athlete to stay hydrated. Dehydration makes the body inefficient at handling blood sugar.

If your athlete has diabetes, he or she will need to understand the interplay of food, exercise, and blood sugar. Eating healthy meals and snacks at regular intervals and monitoring the body's response to food with blood sugar checks is the best way to manage and control diabetes, as each athlete is different. Finally, you'll want to closely coordinate with your health care team, particularly as your athlete grows and becomes more committed to his or her sport.

Celiac Disease

A hereditary autoimmune condition affecting at least 3 million Americans, celiac disease involves an allergic response in the gastrointestinal tract to foods containing gluten, causing damage to the intestinal lining and affecting its ability to absorb nutrients.

Foods containing gluten include wheat, rye, barley, and sometimes oats (when contaminated with wheat in processing), and any foods made with these. Symptoms of celiac disease include chronic diarrhea; abdominal bloating, cramping, and pain; poor weight gain and overall growth; fatigue; anemia; joint pain; low bone density; and irregular menstruation. Chronic diarrhea has classically been the red flag of celiac disease; however, only 35% of those newly diagnosed have it and instead often experience other problems.[33] Because of the wide array of symptoms, the diagnosis of celiac disease may be prolonged or even misdiagnosed. Diagnosis is based on a series of blood tests, intestinal biopsies, the nature and history of a person's symptoms, and genetic predisposition.

Treatment for celiac disease involves the strict avoidance of any foods containing gluten. Instead of eating gluten-containing foods—cereals, breads, pasta—people with the condition should incorporate gluten alternatives—beans, rice, cornmeal, tapioca, potatoes, nuts, quinoa—into their diets. There are many naturally gluten-free foods (fruit, veggies, beef and poultry, eggs, dairy foods), as well as a large number of gluten-free products on the market today, which makes following a gluten-free diet easier than in years past. One remaining threat to those with celiac disease is cross-contamination (which happens when gluten-containing foods touch gluten-free foods), particularly in sports settings where athletes share food and eat at concession stands.

People with celiac disease are at a higher risk for deficiency of certain nutrients, including iron, calcium, and vitamin D, perhaps due to poor absorption of these nutrients in the gut and perhaps from eating too many foods that are low in those nutrients. An estimated 10% to 70% of newly diagnosed individuals have iron-deficiency anemia.[34] Iron supplements and a high-iron, gluten-free diet are required to reestablish normal iron status, which can take up to 18 months to correct.[35]

Calcium and vitamin D are also poorly absorbed in the gastrointestinal tract in people with celiac disease, and osteopenia (lower than normal bone mineral density) or osteoporosis (a more dramatic reduction in bone minerals that results in decreased bone mass and density) occurs in about 10% to 20% of celiac disease cases.[36] At this time, DEXA scans are not recommended for children with uncomplicated celiac disease; however, parents of young female athletes with celiac disease might want to consider that testing, particularly if the athlete's usual food choices are low in calcium and vitamin D. A gluten-free calcium and vitamin D supplement can be helpful, along with high-calcium foods such as fortified orange juice, broccoli, spinach, fish, amaranth, and quinoa.

Be on the lookout for other nutrient deficiencies, such as deficits in vitamin B_{12}, folic acid, zinc, and copper, which may occur in people with celiac disease. Gluten-free products, particularly grains like gluten-free pasta or cereals, may not contain the same level of nutrients found in regular gluten-containing foods. Many grains available on the market are fortified with B vitamins, folate, and iron, but this isn't always the case with gluten-free items. Your best bet is to find alternate grains—amaranth, buckwheat, millet, brown rice, quinoa, sorghum, teff (an African grain used as a flour in gluten-free recipes and products), and wild rice—that are naturally rich in nutrients.

Managing nutrition for the young athlete with celiac disease takes some forethought and planning, but it's not impossible. The goal is to stay on a gluten-free diet, choose the most nutrient-rich options, and avoid cross-contamination so that symptoms are controlled and physical activity isn't interrupted. The long-term goal, of course, is optimal health and prevention of chronic complications associated with celiac disease, such as osteoporosis and anemia.

Food Allergies

Hank, a 13-year-old basketball player, had five bone breaks in 3 years. He was a thin boy and allergic to peanuts, milk, and eggs. After the fifth bone break, Hank's mom sought my input. Because he couldn't eat dairy (and didn't like nondairy substitutes), Hank's diet wasn't delivering important bone nutrients, like calcium, vitamin D, and protein. He had been eating like this for years, but now his participation in sports was magnifying his dietary gaps. Hank needed a nutrition plan that included reliable sources of calcium and vitamin D, while also steering clear of his food allergies. I added soymilk smoothies to his daily menu, found high-protein food sources that he enjoyed (hamburgers and steak), advised a calcium and vitamin D supplemental chew, and started him on a pre-bedtime snack. His energy improved, and he started to gain some weight—and he hasn't had a bone fracture since.

About 6 million children and teens in the United States have food allergies; the most common are to milk, soy, eggs, peanuts, tree nuts, shellfish, fish, and wheat.[37] Management of food allergies involves preventing an allergic reaction by strictly avoiding specific food allergens. In other words, food-allergic athletes should take the food allergen completely out of their diet; a milk allergy means a diet that is strictly dairy-free. Should an allergic reaction occur, treatment might include the use of an antihistamine, steroids, epinephrine, or a combination of these, depending on the type of reaction. Allergic reactions can range from a mild rash and swelling to a life-threatening, full-fledged anaphylactic reaction involving multiple body systems, including the lungs, heart, skin, and gastrointestinal tract.

Multiple food allergies, such as those Hank had, increase the risk for nutrient deficiencies and growth problems because so many foods are eliminated from the diet. Being allergic to milk and wheat, especially, can have a major impact on the nutritional adequacy of your athlete's diet. Poor growth and nutritional deficiencies are more likely in kids who are allergic to cow's milk and those who are allergic to two or more food allergens.[38] With any food allergy, you want to find nutritious food substitutes that will fill in any potential nutrient gaps. For example, using soymilk in lieu of dairy is an ideal swap because the two types of food contain similar amounts of protein, calcium, and vitamin D. Other alternatives to milk exist as well, such as rice milk, nut milks (though not for athletes with a nut allergy), hemp milk, and coconut milk; however, their protein, calcium, and vitamin D content vary considerably. The objective is to find substitutes for the nutrients that allergic athletes may be missing. For instance, if they are allergic to nuts, find other allergen-free protein substitutes such as edamame, other beans, eggs, and dairy. If they can't eat eggs, opt for high-protein alternatives such as nuts, beans, fish, and lean meats. Keeping your eye on filling in the nutrient gaps created by food allergies will preserve the quality of your athlete's diet without compromising his or her nutritional health or athletic performance.

The risk of allergic reaction via cross-contamination increases in situations where many foods are available, such as at a concession stand, or when athletes can share food or touch each other while they're eating. You can help your allergic athletes stay safe and avoid an allergic reaction by teaching them about cross-contamination and how to avoid it (washing their hands, using packaged foods with ingredients labels, not sharing food or touching other athletes who are eating). Read all ingredients labels for food allergens, and if labels aren't available, such as for homemade concession items, avoid them. For most athletes with food allergies, bringing snacks and drinks from home is an easy way to avoid the risk of reaction.

Food and nutrition are key components in recovery, helping to cure the injured body, and, in the case of chronic conditions, supporting body function and health. No matter what obstacles your young athlete is dealing with, from extra weight or broken bones to diabetes or food allergies, participating in sports, and even excelling at them, is completely possible. Of course, if your athlete is not in good health, as in the case of an eating disorder, or if his or her medical condition is not well managed, competitive sports may have to take a back seat until your athlete's overall health is restored.

Notes

1. Nelson FN, Stovitz SD, Thomas M, LaVoi NM, Bauer KW, and Neumark-Sztainer D. "Do youth sports prevent pediatric obesity? A systematic review and commentary." *Curr Sport Med Reports*. 10 (2011): 360–370.
2. Ibid.

3. McHugh MP. "Oversized young athletes: a weighty concern." *Br J Sport Med.* 44 (2010): 45–49.
4. Caine D, Purcell L, and Maffulli N. "The child and adolescent athlete: a review of three potentially serious injuries." *BMC Sports Sci Med Rehabil.* 6 (2014): 22.
5. Torstveit MK and Sundgot-Borgen J. "Are under- and overweight female elite athletes thin and fat? A controlled study." *Med Sci Sports Exerc.* 44 (2012): 949–957.
6. Turocy PS, DePalma BF, Horswill CA, Laquale KM, Martin TJ, Perry AC, Somova MJ, and Utter AC. "National Athletic Trainers' Association position statement: safe weight loss and maintenance practices in sport and exercise." *J Athl Train.* 46 (2011): 322–336.
7. Nelson et al, op. cit., p. 366.
8. Committee on Nutrition and the Council on Sports Medicine and Fitness. "Sports drinks and energy drinks for children and adolescents: are they appropriate?" *Pediatrics.* 127 (2011): 1182–1189.
9. Manore MM. "Weight management in the performance athlete." *Nestle Nutr Inst Workshop Ser.* 75 (2013): 123–133.
10. Werner A, Thiel A, Schneider S, Mayer J, Giel KE, and Zipfel S. "Weight-control behavior and weight concerns in young elite athletes—a systematic review." *J Eating Disord.* 1 (2013): 18.
11. Ibid., p. 8.
12. National Eating Disorders Association. National Eating Disorders Association Toolkit for Coaches and Trainers. http://www.nationaleatingdisorders .org/coach-trainer.
13. Torstveit and Sundgot-Borgen, op. cit., p. 952.
14. National Eating Disorders Association website. www.nationaleatingdisorders .org.
15. Bonci CM, Bonci LJ, Granger LR, Johnson CL, Malina RM, Milne LW, Ryan RR, and Vanderbunt EM. "National Athletic Trainers' Association Position Statement: preventing, detecting, and managing disordered eating in athletes." *J Athl Train.* 43 (2008): 80–108.
16. Youth Sports Injuries Statistics. Stop Sports Injuries. http://www.stopsports injuries.org/media/statistics.aspx.
17. Brenner JS. "Overuse injuries, overtraining, and burnout in child and adolescent athletes." *Pediatrics.* 119 (2007): 1242–1245.
18. Ibid., p. 1243.
19. Ibid., p. 1244.
20. Hoang QB and Mortazavi M. "Pediatric overuse injuries in sport." *Adv Pediatrics.* 59 (2012): 359–383.

21. Ibid., p. 360.
22. Chen Y, Tenforde AS, and Fredericson A. "Update on stress fractures in female athletes: epidemiology, treatment, and prevention." *Curr Rev Musculoskel Med.* 6 (2013): 173–181.
23. Tenforde AS, Sayres LC, Sainani KL, and Fredericson M. "Evaluating the relationship of calcium and vitamin D in the prevention of stress fracture injuries in the young athlete: a review of the literature." *Phys Med Rehab.* 10 (2010): 945–949.
24. Sonneville KR, Gordon CM, Kocher MS, Pierce LM, Ramappa A, and Field AE. "Vitamin D, calcium, and dairy intakes and stress fractures among female adolescents." *JAMA Pediatrics.* 166 (2012): 595–600.
25. U.S. Department of Agriculture and U.S. Department of Health and Human Services. "*Dietary Guidelines for Americans, 2015.*" Available at: http://www.health.gov/dietaryguidelines/2015-scientific-report/PDFs/Scientific-Report-of-the-2015-Dietary-Guidelines-Advisory-Committee.pdf.
26. American Diabetes Association. "Statistics about diabetes." www.diabetes.org/diabetes-basics/statistics/.
27. Robertson K, Riddell MC, Guinhouya BC, Adolfsson P, and Hanas R. "Exercise in children and adolescents with diabetes. ISPAD Clinical Practice Consensus Guidelines 2014 Compendium." *Pediatr Diabetes.* 15 (2014): 203–223.
28. Ibid., p. 206.
29. Ibid., p. 214.
30. Ibid., p. 208.
31. Ibid., p. 214.
32. Ibid., p. 210.
33. Fasano A, Berti I, Gerarduzzi T, Not T, Colletti RB, Drago S, Elitsur Y, Green PH, Guandalini S, Hill ID, Pietzak M, Ventura A, Thorpe M, Kryszak D, Fornaroli F, Wasserman SS, Murray JA, and Horvath K. "Prevalence of celiac disease in at-risk and not-at-risk groups in the United States: a large multicenter study. *Arch Intern Med.* 163 (2003): 286–292.
34. Mancini LA, Trojian T, Mancini AC. "Celiac disease and the athlete." *Curr Sport Med Rep.* 10 (2011): 105–108.
35. Ibid., p. 106.
36. Ibid., p. 107.
37. Sicherer S, Acebal ML, and Sampson HA. Food Allergies. *A Complete Guide for Eating When Your Life Depends on It.* Baltimore: Johns Hopkins Press, 2013.
38. Kirby M and Danner E. "Nutritional deficiencies in children on restricted diets." *Pediatr Clin N Am.* 56 (2009): 1085–1103.

CHAPTER 9

The Special Diet Dilemma

Dieting gets athletes into trouble.
—Nancy Clark, sports nutritionist, athlete, and author

Abby, a top-notch tennis player and a cheerleader in high school, was struggling with extra weight gain. Her coaches had expressed concern, as the surplus pounds were affecting her performance, and they sent her to me for help. Unfortunately, Abby had started dieting over the summer on her own, and she was in the midst of a dangerous cycle of dieting, binge eating, and purging. She was losing control of her healthy diet at night, binging on snack foods and sometimes vomiting afterward. Her "healthy diet" was too restrictive for her high activity level, cutting too deeply into her calorie needs. The end result was intense hunger, food cravings, and binge eating. On top of this, she felt guilty and terrible about herself for "being bad" and breaking her diet. Like many people who diet, Abby would start fresh the next day, but her intense hunger would trigger over-eating at night.

The word *diet* is one of the most confusing terms in the field of nutrition. A diet is what you eat and how you eat it. In other words, your everyday eating, whether it's healthy or unhealthy, is your diet. So *diet* is a descriptor with a wide variety of definitions, and it means different things for different people.

One person's diet could be a representation of the ideal balance of food groups discussed in Chapter 5, eaten evenly throughout the day, while another person's diet might either focus on low-fat foods or on an Atkins-type eating pattern (high fat, no carbs). Still another's diet could mean skipping breakfast.

Dieting, on the other hand, is the act of eating differently for the purpose of changing your body weight or shape, or your health, such as by cutting calories, eliminating certain foods or food groups, or crowding out unhealthy foods by adding healthier fare.

Almost 45 million Americans are dieting each year, and their reasons for doing so are broad.[1] People do it to lose weight, improve their health, reverse medical complications, or fulfill a lifestyle or personal belief. A special diet may be medically necessary, such as the gluten-free diet mandated for celiac disease (see Chapter 8), or it may represent a lifestyle approach, such as a vegetarian diet (discussed below). Some diets are used as a quick fix for the extra weight packed on over the holidays or summer break. Many diets are a flash in the pan—short-lived and promising great benefits, but often offering more risk than reward and rarely resulting in lasting change.

The buzz about diets and dieting can be deafening and is often quite confusing. What do you do when your young athlete says, "I need to cut weight," or "I want to become a vegan"? It's hard to know which diets are safe and which are not, especially for your growing athlete. This chapter gives you the scoop on dieting and explains the benefits and potential dangers of several trendy diets for your young athlete.

Diets, Dieting, and the Young Athlete

A healthy diet is a good thing for young athletes, as it will provide the optimal fuel they need for peak performance, on and off the field. In an ironic twist, detrimental dieting often begins with a switch to healthier eating, like cutting back on sweets or giving up soda. While these are undoubtedly healthy measures, they can morph into an unhealthy cycle of under-eating and under-fueling, or even binging, weight gain, and more dieting. The line between healthy and unhealthy eating is blurred when healthy attempts at crowding out the bad stuff turn into skipping meals, eliminating certain food groups, and significantly slashing calories.

Some athletes believe they need to lose weight to improve their athletic performance—whether that is a reality or not. True, some athletes carry extra weight and could stand to lose a few pounds, but others are fine just the way they are. Also true is the idea that in some sports being leaner optimizes performance. However, this is not the rule for every athlete or every sport, so it's important to take a realistic view. For example, if your athlete comes from a stocky heritage and she's a dancer, it's not likely that she will be able to lose weight and become thin in a way that is healthy. Likewise, athletes who are genetically thin will have difficulty bulking up for the football team. Figuring out the best weight for your athlete's optimal performance is the best approach.

Two important things to remember: (1) Whatever the reason for dieting, it's often a short-term solution that ignores the long-term impact. (2) Research indicates that a concern with and focus on body weight predicts future dieting and disordered eating in teens.[2]

Your Food Attitudes and Your Kids' Eating Behavior

Your children tend to mimic your eating habits from a young age, whether those habits are good or bad. If you skip meals, it's more likely that they will, too. If you are frequently on a diet, chances are that they will go on one at some point, too. And if you are unhappy with your children's weight or shape, it's more likely that they will also be unhappy with it. In a 2010 study of moms and teens, researchers found that teens who had a mom who was worried about the teens' weight were more likely to try to lose weight 5 years later.[3] Furthermore, if you're worried about your children's weight, you may restrict or limit their food or encourage them to diet, either of which may send them down the road of disordered eating.[4]

Dieting is dangerous. And you have the power to influence whether your children adopt healthy or unhealthy eating habits. Get good habits started at a young age and your athletes will be on firmer ground when they are faced with the temptation to diet.

The pressure—from coaches, the media, peers, and even you, perhaps—to be lean and fit and to excel in a sport makes your young athlete more susceptible to dieting. Some young athletes engage in weight-control behaviors despite knowing how important a healthy diet and long-term health are to their sports success.[5] Young athletes who participate in sports that emphasize leanness—such as running, gymnastics, or lightweight rowing—may be more inclined to use unhealthy weight-loss tactics than athletes in other sports, but we need to learn more in this area.[6]

"One of the most common patterns for young athletes is to sleep through breakfast, eat a salad for lunch, try to perform at their sport after school, become light-headed or overly tired, come home starving, overeat, get mad at themselves, get up the next day, and start all over," says Nancy Clark, a registered dietitian, author, and well-known Boston-based sports nutritionist. Instead, Clark encourages athletes to fuel by day and lose weight by night. "Eating less at the end of the day, by knocking off 100 to 200 calories, allows athletes to lose weight while sleeping, not during the day when they're going to school and playing a sport," says Clark. "It's hard to lose weight and have energy to exercise," she warns. "Chip away the calories, a little bit at a time, by eating less after dinner, and ask yourself, 'Do I want to be leaner, or do I want to eat more?'"

Some of the methods young people use to lose weight, such as skipping meals, fasting (going long periods without eating), using meal substitutes such as nutrition shakes, and taking diet pills, laxatives, or diuretics, are considered unhealthy and are associated with an increased risk for disordered eating. You may be surprised to know that over 50% of teen girls and 33% of teen boys use these unhealthy tactics to control or lose weight.[7] The kicker? These methods are associated with *weight gain*, not weight loss.

In a 2012 study of middle school and high school teens, researchers found significant weight gain in both boys and girls over a 10-year period when unhealthy weight loss tactics, especially skipping meals and fasting, were used.[8] While this research wasn't athlete-specific, it speaks to the tendency of teens to use drastic measures to lose weight. And the research is clear on dieting—it backfires.

While eventual weight gain may be one of the complications of dieting, there may be other side effects for your athlete. For one, the association between dieting and disordered eating is real. In a 2006 study, researchers found that teens who engaged in unhealthy dieting practices were more likely to binge eat and use dangerous methods, such as vomiting and laxative abuse, to control their weight 5 years later.[9]

Abby, whose case was cited at the start of the chapter, is an example of what can go wrong when athletes start dieting. Dieting was at the root of her eating problems, which had morphed into a bigger problem—an eating disorder.

Not all athletes will develop an eating disorder just because they go on a diet. But other significant nutritional complications may occur. Desirable levels of nutrients—particularly iron, calcium, and vitamin D, but others as well—may be compromised, especially if the athlete skips meals or cuts foods out of her diet. Eating less means athletes get fewer nutrients during the day, especially if they don't eat alternatives to the foods they're excluding.

Athletes can experience anemia, fatigue, and a higher risk of illness and infection when the daily intake is low in nutrients.[10] Some athletes may see a short-term improvement in performance when they follow a diet, especially if some weight reduction is needed, but the long-term impact of insufficient energy and nutrients to the body may negatively affect athletic performance by lowering oxygen uptake in the muscles and reducing speed.[11]

As you can probably guess, my advice on diets is to stay away from them, because they can lead to cyclical dieting, disordered eating, and eventually even an eating disorder. However, knowledge is power, and the more you know about the effects of dieting and the different diets your athlete may be trying, the better able you will be to monitor your athletes' diet and to intervene when their eating becomes detrimental or even dangerous.

Mainstream Diets: Do They Deliver?

Many of today's popular diets, such as the Atkins diet or the paleo diet, advocate some of the unhealthy weight-control measures described above, such as eliminating certain nutrients (such as carbs) or food groups (such as grains and dairy). Be wary of these diets and suspicious of their promises. Weight loss isn't the be-all and end-all, especially if along the way your athlete incurs fatigue or a nutrient deficiency.

Other diets, such as the Mediterranean diet, feature a balance of nutrients and focus on the healthy qualities of certain nutrients, such as omega-3 fatty acids, which can be a healthful way of eating. Some diets will be risky for your athlete, some will be harmless, and some, such as the vegetarian diets discussed below, will require forethought and planning on your part.

Your athletes may say they're on a particular diet, but they may be making unhealthy modifications to their eating patterns without your knowledge. Keep the lines of communication open, be curious, and be a knowledgeable resource should your athletes inquire about or want to follow a special diet. Sometimes, just helping your athletes set healthy eating patterns, based on the principles outlined in Chapter 5, is the best strategy.

Remember, children and teens are apt to eat food that is accessible. Make healthy items readily available and easy to eat. Teens are more prone to dieting than children, which relates to their developmental stage: teens seek independence, want quick results, and follow the crowd, so get ready for this.

Table 9-1 lists seven of today's most popular diets, including their basic guidelines, and the pros and cons for your athlete. *Note:* The inclusion of a diet in the table does not indicate my endorsement or support of it.

Understanding the Needs of the Vegetarian Athlete

About 4% of American children and teens claim they are vegetarian, according to a 2014 poll by Harris Interactive for the Vegetarian Resource Group (VRG).[12] Specifically, between the ages of 6 and 17, approximately 2% of children and teens say they are vegetarian (eating a diet that excludes meat, fish, and poultry), and 6% say they don't eat meat.[13]

Young athletes who are vegetarian largely cut out animal products—meat, dairy, and eggs—from their diet, although some vegetarian athletes eat dairy, eggs, and fish. For vegetarians, the overall dietary focus is eating an abundance of such plant foods as fruit, vegetables, whole grains, nuts, seeds, and beans. This diet can be a nutritious way to fuel your young athletes, provided it includes wholesome foods and adequate nutrients to

Table 9-1 Characteristics of Popular Diets

Diet	Premise	Nutrition Characteristics	Pros	Cons
Paleo diet (aka caveman diet)	Diet reflects the foods eaten by early man when he first roamed the planet; exercise is emphasized	Fish, lean meats, fruit, nonstarchy veggies, and nuts are in; starchy veggies, dairy foods, grains, and processed foods are out	Slashes processed food and desserts	May be difficult to maintain this diet; nutrients such as calcium, vitamin D, and B vitamins may be low due to elimination of dairy and grains
Macrobiotic diet	Diet emphasizes whole foods, meditation, and relaxed lifestyle	Avoids most animal-derived foods; emphasis on whole grains, fruits, and vegetables	Nutrient-rich foods	Rigid guidelines are difficult to adhere to; nutrient deficiencies, especially vitamin B_{12}, calcium and iron due to missing food groups
New Atkins Diet Revolution	Low carb, high protein diet	Eliminates refined grains; controls portions of fat and healthy carbs; whole grains are off limits for several weeks until weight maintenance phase achieved	Cuts down on excess sweets and refined grains	May be lacking calcium, B vitamins, and potassium; high protein may contribute to heart and kidney disease
Mediterranean diet	Emphasizes healthy fats, including omega-3 fatty acids	Seafood, nuts and legumes, fruits and vegetables, whole grains, olive oil, and red wine in moderation	Heart healthy	Alcohol

Diet	Premise	Nutrition Characteristics	Pros	Cons
Volumetrics	Emphasizes high water content food for their filling effect and low calorie content	Fruits and vegetables	Nutrient-rich food sources; eat to fullness	Requires home-cooking
Raw food diet	Based on belief that cooking food breaks down enzymes and reduces nutritional benefits	Restricts food cooked or heated above 116° to 118°F; food must be raw and vegetarian	Unlimited food intake; focus on fresh produce and avoids processed foods	Lacks nutrients; difficult to maintain; risk of contamination
Zone Diet	Planned to control inflammation in the body	A division of 40%/30%/30% protein, carbs, and fat; diet includes low-fat protein, non-starchy vegetables and fruit, minimal healthy fat sources; low calories	All foods legit, as long as they fit into the 40%/30%/30% balance of foods meal to meal	May be calorie deficient and cause deficiencies of B vitamins, potassium, and calcium; not scientifically proven to benefit athlete performance or recovery

cover the demands of growth and sport.[14] The goals for young athletes who are vegetarian are to achieve normal growth and development, to stay in good health, and to compete to the best of their abilities.

There are several types of vegetarians:

Lacto-vegetarian: One who eats no animal flesh, but does consume milk. The at-risk nutrients for this vegetarian are iron, zinc, and docosahexaenoic acid (DHA).

Lacto-ovo vegetarian: One who eats no animal flesh, but does consume milk and eggs. The nutrients of concern with this diet are iron and zinc.

Pescetarian: One who eats no animal flesh or animal products, but does eat fish. Nutrients of concern include iron, zinc, calcium, and vitamins D and B_{12}.

Vegan: One who does not consume any foods of animal origin. The at-risk nutrients are protein, iron, zinc, DHA, calcium, vitamin D, and vitamin B_{12}.

Flexitarian: One who follows a vegan diet, but occasionally consumes meat, fish, poultry, or dairy. This flexibility allows the requirements for all nutrients to be met with thoughtful planning.

Following a vegetarian diet may lower the risk for heart disease, reduce levels of cholesterol and triglycerides, lower blood pressure, drop the risk of type 2 diabetes, reduce weight, and minimize the risk of certain cancers. These health benefits seem to be related to the increased consumption of plant foods, which are good sources of micronutrients, antioxidants, fiber, and phytochemicals, rather than to the elimination of animal products.[15]

The ability to ward off common colds and other diseases—that is, having a strong immune system—is a compelling reason for some athletes to go vegan. After all, getting sick less translates to fewer training disruptions. Improved immunity is linked to the high micronutrient load associated with vegan diets.[16] Nutrients called antioxidants are, in part, responsible for supporting the immune system, and several nutrients, including beta-carotene, vitamin C, and vitamin E, are powerful antioxidant nutrients. If you want to bump up the antioxidant levels in your athlete's diet and curtail frequent illness, try adding more fruits and vegetables to the diet, particularly the foods that are high in antioxidants: black currants; berries; pomegranate; sour cherries; oranges; kiwi; all colorful vegetables (green, red, orange, yellow, etc.); pistachios; and sesame seeds.

Endangered Nutrients

If your athlete is vegan, or any form of vegetarian, you will need to pay attention to some critical nutrients. Often young athletes ignore this aspect of being vegetarian, but given their age and the nutritional demands of growth and sport, these nutrients are a top priority:

Protein. Protein needs are similar in vegan and non-vegan athletes.[17] Vegans can get protein from grains, vegetables, tofu, beans, nuts, and seeds, but they may have to eat more of these foods to glean the amounts of protein that animal sources can supply. As long as vegan protein sources are varied throughout the day, protein needs, particularly amino acids, should be easy to meet. Occasionally, vegans may use isolated protein powders like pea or soy protein to bump up their overall intake of protein, especially if their whole-food sources are marginal as in the young athlete who won't eat beans, or the teen athlete who drinks low protein milk substitutes. Whole-food sources of protein are ideal. Larger athletes with higher protein needs, such as teen football players, may need a protein powder supplement to meet their daily protein needs while they are on a vegan diet.[18]

Calcium. Calcium is found in certain vegetables, such as bok choy, kale, watercress, and arugula, as well as in nuts, especially almonds, and seeds such as sesame and chia. Because children aged 9 to 18 years need more calcium than at any other time in their life for bone development (1,300 mg per day), seeking out calcium sources and including them routinely in the diet is critical. Other top plant sources of calcium include collard greens, spinach, kidney beans, tofu, calcium-fortified orange juice, calcium-fortified cereals, and alternative milks such as soymilk that are calcium-fortified.

Iron. As you know, young athletes are susceptible to iron deficiency, especially girls, due to iron losses associated with exercise and menstruation. For any athlete, iron deficits can diminish athletic performance. Iron from plant foods is harder to absorb than iron from animal flesh. However, iron absorption can be improved by consuming a vitamin C source, such as citrus juice, along with plant sources of iron. Include quality iron and vitamin C sources daily, such as spinach tossed into a strawberry smoothie, or citrus vinaigrette drizzled atop a kale salad. Top plant sources of iron include spinach, asparagus, chard, broccoli rabe, bok choy, firm or soft tofu, lentils, soybeans, other beans, pumpkin seeds, sesame seeds, raisins, and iron-fortified breakfast cereals.

Beans and grains, while a good source of iron, also contain phytates, which are antioxidant compounds that inhibit the absorption of iron in the body. The best way around them is to eat a vitamin C source when eating beans or grains, which will enhance iron absorption and reduce their inhibitory effects. For example, a pasta meal with white beans and tomatoes promotes iron absorption due to the presence of tomatoes (a vitamin C source) in the meal.

Zinc. The primary source of zinc in the American diet is animal products. Although there are plant sources of zinc, such as beans, whole grains, and nuts, they may not be well absorbed due to their phytate content (see above). For this reason, a vegan athlete's need for sources of zinc is about 50% higher than a non-vegan athlete's.[19] Meeting the zinc requirement from food alone can be a challenge for a vegan athlete, so a multivitamin/multi-mineral supplement may be warranted. Top plant sources of zinc include black beans, other beans, tofu, cashews, bean-based veggie burgers, fortified breakfast cereals, peas, pumpkin seeds, and hemp seeds.

Vitamin B$_{12}$. Deficiencies of vitamin B$_{12}$ can cause anemia and may even lead to permanent central nervous system damage. Vitamin B$_{12}$ is found largely in animal foods, so the vegan athlete will need a reliable source—a fortified food such as nutritional yeast, fortified soy products or cereals, soymilk, B$_{12}$-fortified meat analogues, or a vitamin B$_{12}$ supplement. If your athlete eats dairy and eggs, his or her vitamin B$_{12}$ intake may be fine.

Vitamin D. Most of the fortified food sources of vitamin D are unavailable to vegans who eliminate dairy products and eggs. Of course, athletes who live in a sunny climate year-round and spend time outside without sunscreen may make enough vitamin D in their skin. However, for general health and wellness, a vitamin D supplement is not a bad idea. Aim for at least the Recommended Dietary Allowance (RDA) (600 International Units [IU] per day). Plant food sources of vitamin D include vitamin D–fortified orange juice, mushrooms, soymilk, and some vitamin D–fortified cereals.

DHA. Fatty fish is the richest food source of DHA, so if your athletes are vegan, they may not be getting enough DHA in their diet. The jury is still out on whether athletes should supplement their dietary intake of DHA, but I support routinely including a source of this fatty acid, whether from eating fish twice weekly or taking an algae-based DHA supplement.

Typical Mistakes

"I want to be a vegetarian," said 11-year-old Kayla, an avid volleyball player.

"Do you know what that involves?" I asked Kayla and her mom.

"Yes," said Kayla, "I can eat macaroni and cheese, pizza, and yogurt." Her mom shook her head left and right, and said, "Jill, this is why we are here."

Sometimes young athletes don't understand the variety of foods they must eat in order to be a healthy vegetarian, including beans, green vegetables, tofu, and seeds. These foods alone can make an eager adopter shy away from pursuing a vegetarian diet. Unfortunately, some young athletes forge ahead without the knowledge they need to maximize their health and maintain or even enhance their athletic performance. Here are some of the typical vegetarian mistakes I see, and how to transform them:

1. *Not enough high-quality protein.* Today's parents often confront picky eating, specific food preferences, and easy access to fast food. Young athletes can easily skirt the beans, nuts, seeds, whole grains, and veggies that offer the highest-quality protein for a vegetarian. Instead, they go for plain pasta, potatoes, or an occasional slice of cheese pizza. Low protein intake can cause poor growth and fatigue. Make sure your young athlete gets a high-quality protein at each meal, and try to add a protein source to snacks as well. Table 9-2 lists the vegetarian protein options in the different food groups.

2. *Carb-heavy diet.* Bring on the bread. Oh, and maybe some pasta or rice too. And don't forget the dessert! These are the foods most athletes love, and going vegetarian can further encourage a preference for them. Carbs are a good thing, especially for the athlete, but when we're talking about nutrition, too much can be, well, too much. Don't fall into the starchy-carb habit. Make sure there's a balance of carbs, protein, and fat in your athlete's diet, using the guidelines laid out in Chapters 2 and 5.

3. *Too many processed foods.* Cooking for a vegetarian when everyone else in the family is an omnivore (in other words, eats everything, including meat) can make even the most conscientious cook run out for a frozen dinner, fast food, or carryout. But beware of too many foods

Table 9-2 Vegetarian Protein Options

Grains	Quinoa, amaranth, oats, bulgur, buckwheat, Ezekiel bread *Other whole grains such as bread, crackers, pasta, and brown rice contain a small amount of protein*
Vegetables	Peas, spinach, baked potato, broccoli, Brussels sprouts, corn
Beans	All beans are a good source of protein; try kidney, black, navy, white, pinto, lentils, soybeans (edamame), and dips made from beans, such as hummus; products made from soy, such as tofu and tempeh, are a good source of protein
Nuts and seeds	Almonds, cashews, peanuts, and other nuts; pumpkin seeds, sesame seeds, sunflower seeds, hemp seeds, chia seeds
Nut butters	Peanut butter, soy butter, sunflower butter, and other nut butters
Dairy	Milk, yogurt, Greek yogurt, cheese, cottage cheese, kefir
Dairy alternatives	Soy milk, cheese, and yogurt; hemp milk; oat milk
Egg	Eggs, all types
Meat analogues	Soy hot dog, veggie burger, texturized vegetable protein (TVP), Quorn (mycoprotein)

that come out of boxes and bags. It doesn't matter what kind of vegetarian your athlete is; everyone—young people and adults—should cut back on processed foods.

4. *Limited food variety.* If your athletes are vegetarian, and not adventurous eaters, you may have trouble getting them to eat a healthy variety of foods so that, ultimately, they get a healthy array of nutrients. In general, I don't advise picky eaters to become vegetarians as it makes feeding and eating more difficult. Additionally, you'll want to avoid getting into a rut and always providing the same foods, meals, and snacks. Food variety is your ticket to a healthy vegetarian athlete.

5. *Weight-loss strategy.* Some young athletes adopt a vegetarian diet for the purpose of losing weight. Krista, a high school tennis player whose fitness instructor encouraged her to become a raw vegan (someone who eats only uncooked vegetarian foods), lost weight, mostly muscle mass, and thus her tennis ranking tanked. She became tired early in matches and was on a losing streak. Meanwhile, her obsession with food grew. She was hungry all the time and focused intently on food. She began hoarding large amounts of vegetables and fruit from home

and from the school cafeteria. The school caught up with the hoarding (and stealing), and suspended her. If your young athlete is following a vegetarian diet, and losing weight without needing to, this may be a red flag for disordered eating.

How do you know if going vegan is truly a sign of a dangerous eating behavior? In a 2012 study, researchers found that "semi-vegetarians" (those who ate chicken but avoided meat, for example) were more likely to exhibit disordered eating patterns than true vegans who avoided animal products. They found that semi-vegetarians were motivated by weight loss or weight control, while vegans were motivated by ethical concerns related to animals.[20,21]

It's certainly possible that your athletes are using a vegetarian diet to mask their efforts at weight control; however, look for your answer in the intent behind the food choices. If your athletes are motivated by ethical concerns for animals and are willing to eat a broad range of food and nutrients, it's not likely there is a problem with their eating. However, if your athletes are trying to control their eating or weight by eliminating one or more food groups, or aren't willing to address the gamut of nutrients that are critical for health, or seem preoccupied by food and eating, you have grounds for concerns about the possibility of disordered eating. If this is the case, talk with your athletes about proper eating, and consult with specialized health care providers, such as your physician, registered dietitian/nutritionist, or therapist.

Tips for Feeding Your Vegan Athlete

Don't let your young athletes manage a vegan or vegetarian diet on their own. While the desire to be independent with this diet approach may be strong, most young athletes don't have the knowledge of nutrition to eat properly. Here are some simple tips to keep in mind:

1. *Serve a variety of food each day.* Be willing to explore and experiment with different plant foods, especially those that are packed with nutrition. Include hummus, bean dips, and roasted beans. Don't fear tofu—get creative with stir fry, tofu-enriched smoothies, and breakfast scrambles. Find ways to include dark greens and

other colorful fruits and vegetables every day. Make whole grains your go-to, as these are richer in nutrition than their refined or white-wheat counterparts.

2. *Find a routine dairy source or an alternative.* Whether it be cow's milk, soymilk, hemp milk, or a cheese or yogurt alternative, make sure that each day your athletes get three cups of dairy or a non-dairy alternative that is fortified with calcium and vitamin D. Tap into other foods that are good sources of calcium and vitamin D. Your young athletes' bones depend on it.

3. *Pop in the protein.* Check out Table 9-2 for vegetarian protein sources and include at least one at each meal and with most snacks.

4. *Eat with structure and routine.* Sometimes a vegan diet can be very filling because it is chock-full of fiber. The result? Your young athletes don't "have room" for the calories or range of nutrients they need. You can deal with this by offering frequent meals and snacks at regular intervals, such as every 3 to 4 hours, which will allow your athletes plenty of opportunity to eat without becoming overly full and meanwhile get the calories and nutrients they need.

5. *Details, details—they matter.* Pay attention to the nutrients of concern I outlined earlier, including vitamin B_{12}, zinc, iron, calcium, vitamin D, and DHA. If you can cover these, you will have a healthy vegan athlete.

A healthy diet includes all the nutrients your athlete needs, showcased in a variety of foods, and spaced out evenly throughout the day. This can be accomplished using a vegan diet, a medically prescribed diet, or even some of the mainstream diets available today. What doesn't work in the long run is opting for quick-fix solutions to lose weight or improve appearance, such as cutting out food groups, skipping meals, or using unhealthy practices; these are a recipe for problems with eating and weight later on.

What works well is to crowd out foods that are low-octane fuel sources—sweets, soda, junk-food snacks, and fried foods—and focus on high-octane foods such as whole grains, lean protein, low-fat dairy or non-dairy substitutes, fruits, and veggies. Feed your young athletes regularly, fueling them for the day. Your attitude matters also. You need to view and talk about food as the fuel your athletes need to perform. The focus should be on boosting athletic performance with fuel rather than taking away fuel to change weight or appearance.

Notes

1. Boston Medical Center. "Nutrition and weight management." http://www .bmc.org/nutritionweight/services/weightmanagement.htm.
2. Loth KA, MacLehose R, Bucchianeri M, Crow S, and Neumark-Sztainer D. "Predictors of dieting and disordered eating behaviors from adolescence to young adulthood." *J Adoles Health*. 55 (2014): 705–712.
3. Van den Berg PA, Keery H, Eisenberg M, and Neumark-Sztainer D. "Maternal and adolescent report of mother's weight-related concerns and behaviors: Longitudinal associations with adolescent body dissatisfaction and weight control practices." *J Pediatr Psychol*. 35 (2010): 1093–1102.
4. Scaglioni S, Salvioni M, and Galimberti C. "Influence of parental attitude in the development of children's eating behavior." *Br J Nutr*. 99 (2008): S22–S25.
5. Werner A, Thiel A, Schneider S, Mayer J, Giel KE, and Zipfel S. "Weight-control behavior and weight concerns in young elite athletes—a systematic review." *J Eating Disord*. 1 (2013):18.
6. Ibid.
7. National Eating Disorders Association website. www.nationaleatingdisorders .org.
8. Neumark-Sztainer D, Wall M, Story M, and Standish AR. "Dieting and unhealthy weight control behaviors during adolescence: associations with 10-year changes in body mass index." *J Adolesc Health*. 50 (2012): 80–86.
9. Neumark-Sztainer D, Wall M, Guo J, Story M, Haines J, and Eisenberg M. "Obesity, disordered eating, and eating disorders in a longitudinal study of adolescents: How do dieters fare 5 years later?" *J Am Diet Assoc*. 106 (2006): 559–568.
10. Sundgot-Borgen J, Meyer NL, Lohman TG, Ackland TR, Maughan RJ, Stewart AD, and Muller W. "How to minimize the health risks to athletes who compete in weight-sensitive sports. Review and position statement on behalf of the Ad Hoc Research Working Group on body composition, health, and performance, under the auspices of the IOC Medical Commission." *Br J Sports Med*. 47 (2013): 1012–1022.

11. Ingler F and Sundgot-Borgen J. "Influence of body weight reduction on maximal oxygen uptake in female elite athletes." *Scand J Med Sci Sports*. 1 (1991): 141–146.

12. Casalena N. "How many teens and other youth are vegetarian and vegan? The Vegetarian Resource Group asks in a 2014 national poll." http://www .vrg.org/blog/2014/05/30/how-many-teens-and-other-youth-are-vegetarian -and-vegan-the-vegetarian-resource-group-asks-in-a-2014-national-poll/.

13. Ibid.

14. Craig WJ, Mangels AR, and the American Dietetic Association. "Position of the American Dietetic Association: vegetarian diets." *J Am Diet Assoc*. 109 (2009): 1266–1282.

15. Barr SI and Rideout CA. "Nutritional considerations for vegetarian athletes." *Nutrition*. 20 (2004): 696–703.

16. Craig et al, op. cit.

17. Fuhrman J and Ferreri DM. "Fueling the vegetarian (vegan) athlete." *Curr Sports Med Rep*. 9 (2010): 233–241.

18. Rosenbloom CA and Coleman EJ, eds. *Sports Nutrition: A Practice Manual for Professionals*, 5th ed. Chicago: Academy of Nutrition and Dietetics, 2012.

19. Ibid.

20. Timko CA, Hormes JM, and Chubski J. "Will the real vegetarian please stand up? An investigation of dietary restraint and eating disorder symptoms in vegetarians versus non-vegetarians." *Appetite*. 58 (2012): 982–990.

21. Forestell CA, Spaeth AM, and Kane SA. "To eat or not to eat red meat. A closer look at the relationship between restrained eating and vegetarianism in college females." *Appetite* 58 (2012): 319–325.

CHAPTER 10

Changing the Youth Sports Nutrition Landscape

If you aren't going all the way, why go at all?
—Joe Namath, former National Football League
quarterback

Carol, whose 8-year-old daughter Sarah started playing soccer, found that she was frustrated with the Saturday soccer games. "Every time we finish a game, Sarah is offered a snack I'd rather she not have," she complained. "I'm working hard to help her be more active and eat healthier, but soccer is ruining my best-laid plans."

Head out to a soccer game and you'll find plenty of little hands carrying packaged chips and colorful juice drinks. Go to a baseball game and you can grab hot dogs for lunch or nachos for dinner at the concession stand. And the basketball court can satisfy your desire for salty popcorn and candy. At nearly every sporting venue, from the pool to the field, you will find food everywhere, but not what a young, growing athlete *should* be eating.

Playing a sport is supposed to be a positive influence on kids' and teens' lives. Sports are supposed to help kids and teens become healthier and fitter. But the modern reality of playing a sport is this: the food environment at sports games and practices is often hazardous to your athlete's health.

Children and teens who participate in today's youth sports are surrounded by a food circus. An unhealthy food environment coupled with celebrity endorsements and sponsorships threaten to hijack your athletes' food preferences and choices—even their health. The physical exercise involved in playing a sport improves health, but what was once a healthy endeavor is being challenged and compromised by a food environment that easily negates the benefits a sport grants.

As you have learned throughout this book, nutrition is an important factor for sports performance, yet you wouldn't know it to look at the foods offered at a typical competition. Unhealthy food is alive and well in your athlete's sporting experience.

This chapter summarizes the latest science on the food environment associated with youth sports; explores issues such as marketing, sponsorships, and celebrity endorsements; and lays out what it will take to change this environment for the better. If we want our young athletes to be healthier, stronger, and able to reach their growth and athletic potential, we need to create an environment that makes good nutrition easy—and the norm.

The Big Offenders

Before we talk about how to change the food landscape around youth sports, we first need to discuss what's at play, from the type of food offered to the role of each and every one of us, as stakeholders for change. Sport has the potential (indeed, the responsibility) to exemplify good nutrition.

But the truth is, the world of youth sports has been compromised by unhealthy options, food and beverage marketing, coaches who don't "walk the talk" of healthy eating, parents who take the path of least resistance, and more. The biggest problem is that it's simply too easy for your young athlete to get off-track with nutrition. In a nutshell, healthy eating is the hard choice, not the easy one.

Research tells us that kids who play organized sports are more active, consume a healthier diet, and have fewer weight problems even though they consume more calories than their counterparts who don't play sports.[1] But this good news may turn sour if we don't do something, fast. Recently youth sports have been identified as a potential contributor to childhood obesity; the incidence of childhood weight problems among children and teens playing sports is growing.[2] Among the reasons children aren't becoming fitter or healthier as a result of playing sports are the types of food available to them, food and beverage marketing, venue and team sponsorships, and celebrity endorsements.

High-Calorie Food

Anywhere you find kids and teens playing sports, you can bet there will be concession stands, team snacks, and maybe even food trucks. Most concerning is the discrepancy between what athletes *should* be eating and what they *are* eating at sports venues. Nachos, chili fries, slushies, French fries with cheese dip, candy, and a long list of other junk foods tip the calorie needle so far to the right that burning off those calories becomes next to impossible.

In a recent study of the food available to young baseball players in North Carolina, researchers found that nearly 90% of foods eaten at the ballpark were purchased from the concession stand, where 73% of the items available were considered to be unhealthy. In fact, the study identified 72% of concession snacks as high-calorie, low-nutrient options. More than half of the beverage options were of the sugar-sweetened variety. The researchers concluded that high-calorie snacks and sugary-sweet beverages actually dominated the food environment.[3] Table 10-1 lists the foods typically available at the concession stand and the calorie dent of those foods.

Team snacks brought in by parents aren't much better. Those donuts, orange fishy crackers, and electric-blue juice drinks walk right up to the sideline, usually with an adult hand holding the bag. Why are parents contributing to this unhealthy food landscape? Peer pressure is one reason. Parents feel the pressure from other parents and their own children to pony up junk food on the sidelines and for halftime breaks. The fact that relatively few teams have guidelines for snacks doesn't help the situation.

Table 10-1 Calories Count! Common Concession Stand Foods

Food	Typical Serving Size	Calories per serving (kilojoules (kJ))	Fat (grams per serving)	Sugar (grams per serving)
Soda	12 oz (1 can) (330 mL)	140 (586 kJ)	0	40
Gatorade	20 oz (1 bottle) (592 mL)	130 (544 kJ)	0	35
Hot chocolate	8 oz (237 mL)	150 (628 kJ)	1.5	28
Soft pretzel	1 (62 g)	210 (879 kJ)	2	0
Nachos	¼ cup (30 g) cheese + 20 chips	300 (1255 kJ)	16	3.5
Fritos	1 oz (28 g)	160 (669 kJ)	10	0.5
Popcorn	1 small bag (4 cups) (44 g)	200 (837 kJ)	9	0
Pizza (cheese)	1 large slice (168 g)	275 (1151 kJ)	10	4
Hot dog (no bun)	1 (57 g)	185 (774 kJ)	17	1
Chili fries (French fries with chili topping)	1 serving (170 g)	370 (1548 kJ)	16	2
Potato chips	1 oz (28 g)	160 (669 kJ)	10	0
Slim Jim (beef jerky meat snack)	1 oz stick (28 g)	150 (628 kJ)	13	0
Skittles	1 bag (2.2 oz) (62 g)	250 (1046 kJ)	2.5	47
Sour Punch Straws	1 package (57 g)	210 (879 kJ)	1	26
M & M's	1 package (1.7 oz) (48 g)	240 (1004 kJ)	10	31
Twix	1 package (2 bars) (58 g)	250 (1046 kJ)	12	24
Reese's	1 package (2 pieces)	210 (879 kJ)	13	21
Kit Kat	1 package (1.5 oz) (42 g)	210 (879 kJ)	11	21
Airhead	1 piece (16 g)	60 (251 kJ)	1	9
Oreos	1 package (4 cookies) (1.2 oz or 34 g)	160 (669 kJ)	7	13
Fruit snacks	1 bag (2.25 oz) (63 g)	130 (544 kJ)	0	18
Trail mix	1 package (56 g)	280 (1172 kJ)	18	20
Brownie	1 package (2.2 oz) (62 g)	290 (1213 kJ)	13	24
Chocolate chip cookies	1 large cookie (51 g)	220 (920 kJ)	10	18
Nutri-grain bar	1.3 oz (36 g)	120 (502 kJ)	3	11

Another reason is the time factor. Parents are busy and looking for quick kid-pleasers for snack duty—food that they can pick up on the go and that won't spoil, and items the kids will eat. Unfortunately, that reality has translated to packaged crackers, chips, and desserts. As discussed earlier in this book, young athletes often don't burn the calories these snacks provide; they eat more than they've worked off, leaving them in a state of calorie surplus.

In fact, your athlete may not be burning as many calories playing sports as you may think. One study estimated that young athletes engaged in only about 30 minutes of moderate to vigorous activity when participating in their organized sport and spent about 52% of the practice or competition in sedentary or light-intensity activities.[4] The actual physical activity your athlete gets will vary depending on the sport. A 2011 study looked at soccer, baseball, and softball for kids aged 7 to 14 years and found the average amount of physical activity for all three sports was about 45 minutes (which was only 46% of the time allotted for practice).[5] The notion that kids who play sports are burning lots of calories, allowing some leeway in the eating department, appears to be largely a fantasy.

In the long run, one has to question how these unhealthy foods influence your athlete's food choices and preferences. It isn't hard to imagine the answer, especially when we look at other areas of childhood nutrition research. We know that young people choose food that tastes good, and food manufacturers have mastered the art of making less-than-healthy food taste great.[6] Advertisements for food are known to shape the food preferences of kids and teens and to influence their purchases. Frequent exposure to food, from seeing it to tasting it, contributes to a preference and desire for that particular food.[7] The more kids see, taste, and hear about unhealthy food items, the more likely they are to eat, choose, and like them.

Food Marketing, Endorsements, and Sponsorships

If the presence of unhealthy food isn't enough to derail what your athletes eat, the spell woven by advertising and marketing surely keeps it in the forefront of their minds. In general, most parents rate the media and food companies as a negative influence on their kids' eating habits. They feel that the media encourage their kids to want to buy certain food products, encourage bad eating habits, and influence their preference for junk food.[8] It isn't just the kids who are influenced by advertising, though. Parents also perceive food products to be more nutritious when celebrities endorse them—even when they are obviously high in calories and low in nutrients.[9]

Popular sports celebrities like LeBron James and Peyton Manning, who offer the most endorsements for high-calorie, nutrient-poor foods, according to *Bloomberg Businessweek*'s 2010 Power 100 rankings, endorse less-than-healthy foods, leading young athletes to pay more attention to them and to ask parents to buy the celebrity-sponsored products.[10] In a 2013 study, 24% of celebrity endorsements were for food products, and 79% of those were for unhealthy food items. Of the beverages that had athlete endorsements, 93% of them contained calories from added sugar.[11]

Food manufacturers commonly sponsor sports, from little league to local high school sports, helping defray the costs of team uniforms or the overhead associated with running sports programs. Even sponsorships can influence kids and their purchasing decisions. In a 2011 Australian study of children aged 10 to 14 years, investigators found that kids were able to recall the sponsors of their sports clubs; 10- and 11-years-old were more likely to think about the sponsor when buying something to eat or drink, wanted to pay them back for their sponsorship, and thought they were "cool."[12] Sponsors also use rewards for sports performance such as vouchers or gift certificates for a food or beverage product, which has been shown to increase kids' preference for the company and the food after receiving them.[13] Clearly, sponsorships and rewards help mold the food choices and eating patterns of young athletes.

Role Models, Gatekeepers, and Stakeholders

When my older daughters were just starting to play soccer, our town team had a rule about soccer snacks: orange slices and water only. Little did I know how much I would appreciate that modest snack policy, because when my younger children played soccer in later years, I watched the snacks at halftime morph into something very different: cookie packs, cheesy crackers, chips, and donuts, accompanied by a sweet drink. I recall that one mom, who had forgotten that she was on snack duty, sent the whole team to the concession stand and allowed them to buy two items. Most of the kids walked away with a candy bar and a bag of chips. I made my daughter skip the snack. She definitely thought I was a party pooper, but I just couldn't let half a candy bar wipe out all the good she had gained from that day's exercise.

Unhealthy snacks at sports practices and competitions have become the norm rather than the exception—it's a hard and difficult truth. Somehow we've let nutrition slide down the priority list. Adults are the role models, gatekeepers, and stakeholders of nutrition for youth sports. Instead of a message that encourages healthy eating, young athletes are getting a very different idea: "It doesn't matter what you eat."

But here's where it gets a little crazy. You and I and everyone else involved in youth sports know the truth—food and eating do matter. But many adults are caught up in what's happening today, surviving from one practice to the next, and not looking past the next competitive event. Undoubtedly, encouraging young athletes to eat for sport (read: eat healthy food) begins with responsible modeling on the part of the adults in their lives. Let's look at how important it is to be a role model, gatekeeper, and stakeholder in youth sports nutrition.

Role Model. Actions speak louder than words. While parents acknowledge that healthy food is important for their young athletes, for many it's not a priority—at least this is what the research says. Few parents make attempts to change the food landscape at sports venues, according to a 2012 survey.[14] Wanting and hoping for healthier food at sporting events does little to make it a reality.

There are glimmers of hope on the horizon, though, with an uprising of activism from parents who are looking to change the snacking culture in sports. These activists have the right idea, but we need bigger, system-wide changes. No doubt parents who make changes for the betterment of all athletes are powerful role models, not only for their own children, but for other athletes as well.

On the home front, your kids will follow your lead, especially with regard to nutrition. If you opt for the sub sandwich and extra-large soda while watching your child in the stands or skip eating altogether, your athlete may want to do the same. The food you eat and how you eat it imprints your athlete for a lifetime. The emphasis you place on good nutrition also helps direct your athlete to healthy eating. In other words, your athlete is likely to grow up preferring the foods that anchored his or her childhood.

Coaches are role models too. While the ideal coach exercises, eats a well-balanced meal, and embodies a healthy lifestyle, some coaches don't set this example. They may eat poorly and not partake in regular exercise. They may focus on the sport itself but miss the whole picture, such as how nutrition and a healthy lifestyle enhance the sporting experience, and how their own behaviors influence their athlete's choices. Coaches can be great role models simply by showing young athletes how to eat, hydrate, and live a healthy life through their actions and words.

Gatekeeper. Being a nutrition gatekeeper means you are regulating the types of food available to your athlete, such as the food that comes into your home and what you order when eating out. Being good at this isn't easy. It means you have to say no to your athlete sometimes. It means you have to speak out for change when nobody else seems to want it. It means you may have to make an unpopular decision. It takes a lot of moxie to buck the system of junk-food snacks at the concession stand and on the sidelines. But it's worth it.

Time is a real barrier too. The day-to-day pressures of too much to do and too little time make opting for quick food solutions, which may not be the healthiest, a reality. Games or practices that are scheduled during mealtime throw a monkey wrench into the evening, leading some parents to swing through the drive-through or patronize the concession stand. Despite these real obstacles, you are still the decision maker when it comes to what is in the fridge and pantry. You are still the primary influence over what your athlete eats when she's out. And you are the one who pulls out the wallet and pays for what gets supplied to the team when you are on snack duty. You are a powerful gatekeeper.

Coaches, too, set guidelines for acceptable snacks and can mold the standard of eating for young athletes. Parents and coaches are a powerful force when they partner to beat down the barriers, which make it difficult for healthy food options to be the norm. Truly, if the food environment were better, it would be so much easier to feed our young athletes—and we'd all feel a lot better about how they are eating.

Stakeholder. We are all stakeholders with a vested interest in raising healthy athletes. We are all interested in having sports participation be a benefit for our youth and a positive influence on their health and well-being. We can change the food environment in youth sports with a good policy. Families can set a policy of "only healthy food when playing sports"; teams can outline appropriate snack foods, and league leaders can standardize healthy food options at concessions and regulate food marketing and sponsorships.

Parents are warming up to wanting to make significant changes in the sports food landscape. In a 2013 survey, 75% of parents were in support of introducing policies to curb unhealthy food and beverages in children's sports, including alternative funding models in which sponsors forgo visible branding.[15] Adults need to be the change-makers here, not the kids. It's time to take action!

Bucking the System

Changing the food culture in youth sports isn't easy, but doing nothing only endorses it and heightens the health risks for all young athletes. The beginning quotation in this chapter inquires, "If you aren't going all the way, why go at all?" In other words, if you have children who are athletes, have invested your time and money in their athletic endeavors, and want to support them in every way, why *wouldn't* you want the environment they play in to be as healthy as possible? Here are some ideas and supportive materials that can help you make healthy changes happen system-wide.

Parents

You may be asking yourself, "What can *I* do?" The answer is: a lot! Remember, the squeaky wheel gets the grease, and this holds true when it comes to the food available to your young athlete. Here are a few things you can put in place right now:

- Be vocal and ask for what you want. If you want to affect a change in what, if any, snacks are offered at practices or competitions, let it be known. Sally Kuzemchak, RD, calls this "snacktivism"; she offers ideas on her website, Real Mom Nutrition, about how to be a "snacktivist." Warning: Don't be that parent who whines about snacks unless you've made a reasonable suggestion for something different. Discuss potential changes with the coach and talk with other parents. Use this sample letter (see box) to get things started, tweaking it as needed to reflect your style.

Sample Note to Parents about Snacks

Dear Parents,

I am _____'s parent, and I am writing to get feedback from you for our snack policy this season.

Team parents usually have the job of bringing snacks for the players to eat during or after the game is over. This snack is meant to help rehydrate our athletes, replenish their energy, and replace the nutrients they may lose from sweating. We all know that the best snack for young athletes who play for an hour or more is fruit and water. Those athletes playing for an hour or less really don't need food—they just need water and a healthy meal when they get home.

Over the years, sugary drinks, sweets, and packaged foods have become the norm as game snacks. Coach _____ and I are concerned about this because it doesn't help our children reap the benefits of being active in a sport and may even derail their performance and overall healthy eating.

We wanted to bring attention to this matter before the season starts so that we can have a united policy in place. We welcome your opinion on this matter. Would you prefer to have fruit and water as our team snack, or water only? If the decision is made for fruit and water, there will be a snack schedule forthcoming. Thanks for your input!

- Make your own family sports nutrition policy. When it comes to what and when your athlete eats, you set the policy. Aim to have regular meals every day, and encourage your athlete to eat them. Offer healthy snacks both on and off the field, and take the opportunity to explain why they are important. I like the "only healthy fuel for athletes" mantra. Avoid energy drinks and other questionable supplements, and adopt a water-only rule, especially if your athlete is exercising for less than an hour. Stay away from packaged snacks and sweets as they don't build energy and may even be energy-depleting. Having your own sports food policy sets the tone that food choice and eating are important, especially for an athlete.

- Rally your troops. There is strength in numbers, so get other parents of young athletes who are also concerned about the food environment on board with you. Together you can make a difference.

Coaches

Coaches get a better athlete to work with when he or she is fueled with good food. It makes success easier for both athlete and coach, and ensures that the rewards of athletic improvement and success will be tangible. All coaches should work with their athletes' parents to establish communication and guidelines about food, at both practices and competitions. This may require some up-front discussion and reinforcement along the way. A snack policy can outline the team philosophy, comment on the use of food and other incentives as a reward, and offer a list of acceptable snack foods for the athlete.

Coaches can also discuss general nutrition principles with their athletes, either on their own, or by bringing in an expert in the field of sports nutrition. Often young athletes will be more open to nutrition messages from their coaches than to suggestions from their parents. Just make sure coaches have accurate information. Daily reminders from the coach to eat a pre-load snack or meal, recover with nutritious food, and drink adequately send the message that nutrition for sport is important.

I've included a basic snack policy here for the younger athlete (see box), but feel free to adjust it based on the athlete's age and sport. For example, a snack policy for older athletes may outline acceptable snacks with which to pre-load and recover, and items to stay away from, such as candy and fried food. Since older athletes tend to bring their own snacks, the snack policy should reflect guidelines for choosing what to eat, and when.

Sample Snack Policy for Teams

The following is a sample snack policy for your team. Feel free to adjust it to reflect what makes sense for your team and circumstances:

Hello, everyone!

It's time to talk about snacks this season! Our coach has asked me to organize the snacks, but with a change. We are returning to the days of simplicity—for example, orange slices and water—and here's why: we want our kids to burn off energy through their sport, not take in more! We can do that by cutting out the packaged foods, sugary snacks, and sweet drinks that offer our kids more calories than they need after exercising.

Here's our new proposed snack policy for the season:

Kids: Bring your own water to the game. Please keep it to water *only*. Young athletes don't need sugary drinks at all, and a sports drink is really for the athlete who is running hard for more than an hour.

Parents: Share the responsibility of bringing fresh fruit for a snack. You can bring any fresh fruit you'd like, just make sure it's washed and ready for those little hands to grab. Small boxes of dried fruit such as raisins are fine, too. No fruit snacks, roll-ups, or fruit chews (they contain added sugar).

Here are some ideas: orange slices, apple slices, watermelon wedges, berries in a small cup, bunches of grapes, cantaloupe chunks, mixed chopped fruit in a small cup, fruit kabobs, and whole fruit such as bananas, peaches, or pears. If your child won't eat fruit, please bring your own snack and serve it off the field.

This snack policy makes it easy on you and healthy for our kids. It's also less expensive, cleaner, and will contribute to your child's healthy eating for the day, not take away from it. You'll also be more likely to have a hungry child when you return home for mealtime.

If you have any questions about this new snack policy, please let me or the coach know.

Thanks!

Sports League Leaders

Leaders in youth sports have the unique (and difficult) job of balancing the books, garnering funds through fundraising, and moving large sports organizations forward. Yet, as with vending machines and bake sales at schools, many sports organizations are selling and marketing food and beverages to make money for the organization. They allow soda give-aways on the premises, ice cream trucks, and more.

This practice sends the wrong message to our young athletes—essentially that it's okay to trade a profit for their health. There are many ways to make money for your organization, and it doesn't have to involve the sale of unhealthy food. Leagues can sell T-shirts, buttons, hats, and bumper stickers or host a bike-a-thon, swim-a-thon, or other sports-oriented fundraiser. It just takes a little bit of imagination and creativity. And creating a healthy concession stand is easy (see box).

Healthy Concession Stands

Sales at concession stands don't have to showcase candy bars and chips. There are plenty of easy-to-prepare items that will encourage healthy fueling. Get creative and try downsizing the junk and upsizing healthy fuel with these items:

- Fresh, whole fruit
- Low-fat yogurt
- Homemade granola
- Apple slices and peanut butter packs
- Waffle cones filled with fresh chopped fruit
- Veggie cups (fill the bottom of a clear cup with ranch dressing and stand veggie sticks upright)
- Fruit-salad cups
- All-fruit popsicles
- Fruit smoothies
- Frozen grapes or mango chunks
- Large wedges of watermelon
- Hard-boiled egg
- Fruit and cheese kabobs
- Hummus cups and veggie chips

- Guacamole cups and fresh veggies or SunChips
- Prepackaged pita chips and hummus
- Trail mix
- Mozzarella cheese sticks
- Cheddar cheese blocks
- Plain popcorn
- Animal crackers
- Fig Newtons
- Mini-bagel sandwiches (fill with deli cheese, meat, or nut butter and jam)
- Bagels and cream cheese
- Granola bars (with less than 10 grams of sugar per serving)
- Assorted nuts (prepackaged)
- Peanut butter and jelly sandwiches
- Cheese and crackers
- Chocolate milk
- Dried fruit, such as raisins

League authorities may oversee concession stands, general policies about food and beverage marketing, team sponsorships, and fundraising. There are many ways in which sports leaders can spearhead change for the better. Leaders can institute a policy on appropriate food, limiting the sale of unhealthy food items, placing healthy food front and center, and making it affordable. They can create a marketing-free zone at fields and arenas, turning down ads that sell soda and other unhealthy food. They can also banish posters of athletes endorsing food and drinks, discourage free giveaways of unhealthy food and beverages, and be choosy about which pop-up food trucks they allow on site. Finally, league officials may provide links to reputable nutrition information on their website; an increasing number of national leagues and organizations offer nutrition information for their regional and local affiliates.

Don't let today's junk food–filled sports landscape ruin your athlete's healthy diet. Take a stand! Get involved! The food landscape around sports is a culture. You won't change it just by fighting the home-front battle with your athletes, demanding that they eat this and not that. That just sets a negative tone for your own relationship. While you can—and should—

have guidelines and boundaries about healthy and unhealthy food, these will be much easier for your athletes to adhere to when the food environment makes healthy eating easy and the norm. If you want your athletes to reap the benefits of nutrition, you have to work to change the culture of food in sports.

Notes

1. Tomlin DL, Clarke SK, Day M, McKay HA and Naylor P. "Sports drink consumption and diet of children involved in organized sport." *J Int Soc Sport Nutr.* 10 (2013): 38.
2. Nelson TF, Stovitz SD, Thomas M, LaVoi NM, Bauer KW, and Neumark-Sztainer D. "Do youth sports prevent pediatric obesity? A systematic review and commentary." *Curr Sports Med Rep.* 10 (2011): 360–370.
3. Irby MB, Drury-Brown M, and Skelton JA. "The food environment of youth baseball." *Child Obes.* 10 (2014): 260–265.
4. Wickel EE and Eisenmann JC. "Contribution of youth sport to total daily physical activity among 6- to 12-yr-old boys." *Med Sci Sport Exerc.* 39 (2007): 1493–1500.
5. Leek D, Carlson JA, Cain KL, Henrichon S, Rosenberg D, Patrick K, and Sallis JF. "Physical activity during youth sports practices." *Arch Pediatr Adolesc Med.* 165 (2011): 294–299.
6. Moss M. "The extraordinary science of addictive junk food." *New York Times Magazine.* http://www.nytimes.com/2013/02/24/magazine/the-extraordinary-science-of-junk-food.html?pagewanted=all.
7. Birch LL and Fisher JO. "Development of eating behaviors among children and adolescents." *Pediatrics.* 101 (1998): 539–549.
8. Harris JL, Milici FF, Sarda V, and Schwartz MB. "Food marketing to children and adolescents: What do parents think?" Yale Rudd Center for Food Policy and Obesity. http://www.yaleruddcenter.org/resources/upload/docs/what/reports/Rudd_Report_Parents_Survey_Food_Marketing_2012.pdf.
9. Dixon H, Scully M, Wakefield M, Kelly B, and Chapman K. "Parent's responses to nutrient claims and sports celebrity endorsements on energy-dense and nutrient-poor foods: an experimental study." *Publ Health Nutr.* 14 (2011): 1071–1079.
10. Ibid.
11. Bragg MA, Yanamadala S, Roberto CA, Harris JL, and Brownell KD. "Athlete endorsements in food marketing." *Pediatrics.* 132 (2013): 805–810.

12. Kelly B, Baur LA, Bauman AE, King L, Chapman K, and Smith BJ. "'Food company sponsors are kind, generous and cool': (mis)conceptions of junior sports players." *Int J Behav Nutr Phys Act.* 8 (2011): 95.
13. Ibid.
14. Thomas M, Nelson TF, Harwood E, and Neumark-Sztainer D. "Exploring parent perceptions of the food environment in youth sport." *J Nutr Educ Behav.* 44 (2012):365–371.
15. Kelly B, Baur LA, Bauman AE, King L, Chapman K, and Smith BJ. "Views of parents and children on limiting unhealthy food, drink and alcohol sponsorship of elite and children's sports." *Publ Health Nutr.* 16 (2013): 130–135.

RESOURCES

Books

American Dietetic Association's Complete Food and Nutrition Guide, 4th ed., by Roberta Larson Duyff. Thornwood, NY: Houghton Mifflin Harcourt, 2012.

Fearless Feeding: How to Raise Healthy Eaters from High Chair to High School, by Jill Castle and Maryann Jacobsen. New York: Jossey-Bass, 2013.

Fueling the Teen Machine, by Ellen Shanley and Colleen Thompson. Boulder, CO: Bull Publishing Company, 2010.

How to Teach Nutrition to Kids, 4th ed., by Connie Evers. Portland, OR: Twenty Four Carrot Press, 2012.

Intuitive Eating, by Evelyn Tribole and Elyse Reisch. New York: St. Martin's Griffin, 2003.

Mindless Eating: Why We Eat More than We Think, by Brian Wansink. New York: Bantam, 2010.

Nancy Clark's Sports Nutrition Guidebook, by Nancy Clark. Champaign, IL: Human Kinetics, 2013.

Slim by Design: Mindless Eating Solutions for Everyday Life. by Brian Wansink. New York: William Morrow, 2014.

The Teen Eating Manifesto: Ten Essential Steps to Losing Weight, Looking Great, and Getting Healthy, by Lisa Stollman. Toronto: Lisa Stollman/Nirvana Press, 2012.

Cookbooks

Cooking Light: Dinnertime Survival Guide: Feed Your Family. Save Your Sanity, by Sally Kuzemchak and the editors of Cooking Light magazine. Birmingham, AL: Oxmoor House, 2014.

Cooking Light: Fresh Food Fast, Weeknight Meals, by the Editors of Cooking Light Magazine. Birmingham, AL: Oxmoor House, 2010.

Cooking Light: Real Family Food: Simple and Easy Recipes Your Whole Family Will Love, by the editors of Cooking Light magazine. Birmingham, AL: Oxmoor House, 2012.

Cooking Light: Slow Cooker: 57 Essential Recipes to Eat Smart, Be Fit, Live Well, by the editors of Cooking Light magazine. Birmingham, AL: Oxmoor House, 2006.

Don't Panic—Dinner's in the Freezer: Great Tasting Meals You Can Make Ahead, by Susie Martinez, Vanda Howell, and Bonnie Garcia. Ada, MI: Revell Publishing, 2005.

No Whine with Dinner, by Liz Weiss and Janice Bissex. Melrose, MA: M3 Press, 2011.

SOS! The Six O'Clock Scramble to the Rescue: Earth-Friendly, Kid-Pleasing Dinners for Busy Families, by Aviva Goldfarb. New York: St. Martin's Griffin, 2011.

The Barefoot Contessa Cookbooks, by Ina Garten. New York: Clarkson Potter, various years.

The Best Lunch Box Ever: Ideas and Recipes for School Lunches Kids Will Love, by Katie Sullivan Morford. San Francisco: Chronicle Books, 2013.

The Slim Down South Cookbook: Eating Well and Living Healthy in the Land of Biscuits and Bacon, by Carolyn O'Neil and Southern Living. Birmingham, AL: Oxmoor House, 2013.

Websites

www.Healthychildren.org, from the American Academy of Pediatrics.

www.JusttheRightByte.com, my blog via Jillcastle.com.

www.Kidseatright.org, nutrition for kids from the Academy of Nutrition and Dietetics.

www.Kidshealth.org, kids' health and parenting from Nemours.

www.Kids.usa.gov, health for kids K–5th grade.

www.Momsteam.com, the trusted source for sports parents.

www.Nationaleatingdisorders.org, National Eating Disorders Association.

www.Nays.org, National Alliance for Youth Sports.

www.Realmomnutrition.com, Snacktivism blog.

www.Scandpg.org, Sports, Cardiovascular and Nutrition Group.

www.Sikids.com, Sports Illustrated Kids.

www.Teamnutrition.usda.gov, from the U.S. Department of Agriculture's Food and Nutrition Services.

www.Teenshealth.org, teens' health and parenting from Nemours.

www.vrg.org, Vegetarian Resource Group

INDEX